The Bondage Playbook

Quarto.com

© 2025 Quarto Publishing Group USA Inc.

First Published in 2025 by Fair Winds Press, an imprint of The Quarto Group, 100 Cummings Center, Suite 265-D, Beverly, MA 01915, USA.
T (978) 282-9590 F (978) 283-2742

All rights reserved. No part of this book may be reproduced in any form without written permission of the copyright owners. All images in this book have been reproduced with the knowledge and prior consent of the artists concerned, and no responsibility is accepted by producer, publisher, or printer for any infringement of copyright or otherwise, arising from the contents of this publication. Every effort has been made to ensure that credits accurately comply with the information supplied. We apologize for any inaccuracies that may have occurred and will resolve inaccurate or missing information in a subsequent reprinting of the book.

Fair Winds Press titles are also available at discount for retail, wholesale, promotional, and bulk purchase. For details, contact the Special Sales Manager by email at specialsales@quarto.com or by mail at The Quarto Group, Attn: Special Sales Manager, 100 Cummings Center, Suite 265-D, Beverly, MA 01915, USA.

29 28 27 26 25   1 2 3 4 5

ISBN: 978-0-7603-9640-7

Digital edition published in 2025
eISBN: 978-0-7603-9641-4

Library of Congress Cataloging-in-Publication Data available.

This content in this book was originally published under the title *Bondage Basics* by Lord Morpheous (Quiver Press 2015).

Compiled and edited by Jill Hamilton
Design: Quarto Design Team
Cover Image: Mark-Antoine Thibodeau Breault
Illustration: Mark-Antoine Thibodeau Breault

Printed in Hong Kong

The information in this book is for educational purposes only. Any type of sexual activity should be consensual.

The Bondage Playbook

31 Must-Know Knots and Ties for Bondage Beginners

The Editors of Quiver Books

Contents

Introduction: Bondage 101 7
    The Vocabulary of Bondage 10
    Communication 12
    Safety 14
    The Equipment 15
    Bondage Dos and Don'ts 17

CHAPTER 1:
BASIC KNOTS

Bula Bula 20
Lark's Head Knot (also known as the Cow Hitch) 23
Munter Hitch 24
Sommerville Bowline 27
Joining Rope 28
Wrists Behind 31
Two-Column Tie 32
Basic Hair Tie 35
Crossed Wrists Tie 36
DIY Necktie Sex Harness 41

CHAPTER 2:
THE TIES

Beginner Hair Tie with Braid	46
Advanced Hair Tie	50
Kneeling Two-Column Leg Tie	53
The Arm Binder	56
The Broad Chest Harness	61
Basic Futo	64
Ladder Tie	69
Asymmetric Broad Chest Tie	72
Self-Serve Chest Tie	77

CHAPTER 3:
TAKING IT FURTHER

Finger Tie	82
Toe Tie	87
Simple Chest Harness	90
Simple Chest Harness with Wrist Capture	95
Elevated Chest Harness	98
Simple Hip Harness and Leg Weave	103
Beginner Sex Harness Hip Tie	106
The Infinity	111
Karada	114
Ass Opener	119
Trucker's Hitch	121
Rope Corset	124

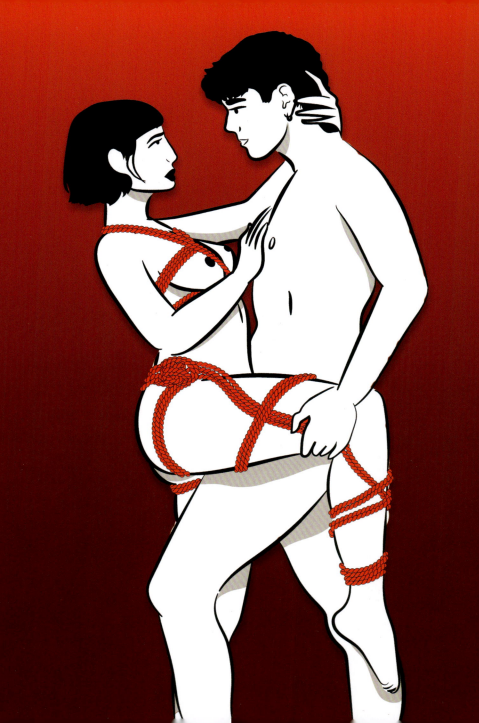

INTRODUCTION:
Bondage 101

Welcome! You have either bravely picked up this book at a bookstore or clicked "buy" online, so you're already at least curious about rope bondage. Whether you're a beginner or looking to expand your rope-wielding horizons, this book has plenty to keep you and your partner tied up with all kinds of adventures.

But first, what even is bondage?

Bondage is tying up or restraining a sexual partner. In this book, we'll be talking mostly about rope bondage. But bondage can be something as simple as pinning your partner's hands down during sex or busting out the handcuffs during role play. Bondage can be a part of sex and/or BDSM—which stands for bondage, discipline, dominance, and submission—but doesn't necessarily have to be. For some people it's all about the sex; others are into it for the Dom-sub dynamic or practice bondage as an art form.

There's pleasure to be had for both the person tying ("the rigger") and the one being tied ("the rope bunny"). For the bunny, it's a chance to totally submit control, leaving them free to get out of their head and just react to the sensations. For some people, that's enough; they just want to enjoy the relaxing headspace that bondage puts them in and don't want any extra stimulation. Others want an intense psychological and physical sexual experience.

For the rigger, there's a rush to having control over someone else's pleasure and watching them submit completely. It can also be a way to express themselves creatively. A rigger might create an intricate design over their bunny's entire torso or use the rope to accentuate a particularly sexy part of their partner's body.

Rope bondage can also serve a practical purpose in BDSM scenes. A harness can guide someone into position. Finger or toe bondage can keep a service-oriented slave in the correct mindset to serve the Dom. A simple rope chastity belt can remind a submissive who they belong to while they're at work.

The act of one person tying up another focuses both people's attention on what's happening in the moment. With sex—and life, for that matter—mindfulness makes the experience feel more intimate and meaningful.

You get to figure out what does it for you. You might want a rough experience like being hog-tied, flogged, and verbally humiliated. Or you might just enjoy the feeling of being fully attended to by having your fingers, hands, feet, or body festooned with colored wool. Up to you. As long as you have enthusiastic consent on both sides, you can go as deep as you want.

How to Use This Book

This book will give you the basics for playing with bondage. You'll get lots of bondage wisdom, including how to talk to a partner, what sort of equipment to use, and how to be safe while tying each other up.

You'll learn the vocab of bondage, the pros and cons of various materials for binding, guidelines for creating good aftercare, and how to build a great bondage kit.

Once you've grasped the basics, you can move on to the good stuff. This book has 31 different knots and ties for your tying pleasure. You'll get the essential starter ties, including how to attach two ropes together, simple knots to finish off an end, and ways to attach a body part to something else. After that, you'll learn ties for specific areas of the body, including how to bind a hand, how to create an intricate binding for a chest, and how to fashion a hip harness to lead a partner exactly where you want them to go.

Once you master the foundational elements, you can mix and match as you please. Want to tie a partner's ankles to the chair legs and their wrists behind them? Sure. A hip harness/chest binding combo for a full-body look? Why not? Or freeform something by getting into your favorite sex position, then adding some ties to it. With this book, you'll have the skills to make it happen. If you have enthusiastic mutual consent and your safety practices are up and running, go ahead and do whatever you damn well please.

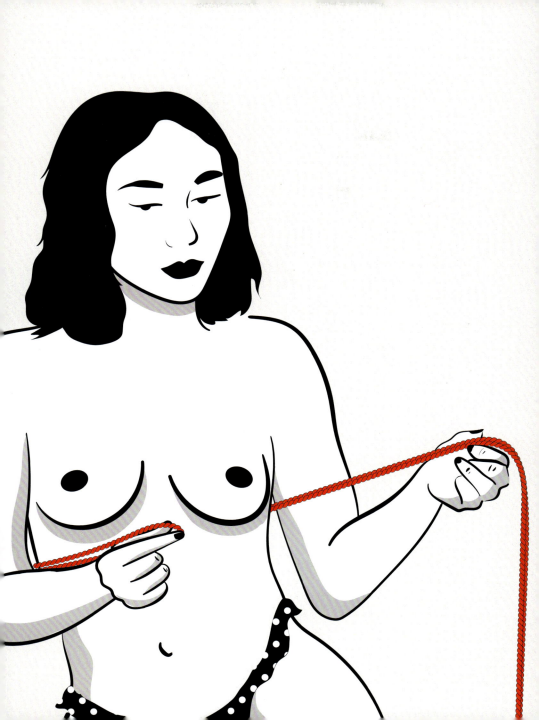

The Vocabulary of Bondage

Before we continue, here's a quick vocabulary list to help you get comfortable using your words:

Aftercare: The physical and mental support given to a submissive by the dominant partner(s) after BDSM play.

Bondage: The practice of tying or restraining a person, most commonly so that they are immobile. A whole host of materials can be used, but rope is the most common.

Bottom: A person who plays a submissive role when required. A bottom may not naturally be a submissive but takes the role in a particular scene if no other submissive is present.

Collaring: To engage in a committed, long-term dominant-submissive relationship. The dominant may place a collar upon the submissive during a special ceremony.

Consent: The most important concept in all of BDSM, this is affirmative permission given in sound mind.

Daddy: A person who takes on the role of a dominant to one or more submissives. This role is nurturing and loving, and may involve education and emotional support as well as general dominant activities.

Dominant (or Dom): A person who likes to be sexually dominant and takes on a role of power or authority over submissives in a power exchange. The dominant is generally in control of a scene with others and calls the shots.

Domme: A female dominant, or a professional dominatrix. A domme may provide nonsexual dominant services to clients.

Hard limits: The lines over which a person will not cross and does not want to approach too closely.

Master/Mistress: A person who lives the BDSM lifestyle 24/7 and has committed to dominating a slave in a total power exchange (TPE).

RACK: An abbreviation for "risk-aware consensual kink," a code of conduct in the BDSM community that is very much adhered to.

Rigger: A universal term for someone who likes to tie up others.

Rope bunny: A person who is into being tied up or restrained by rope. Bunnies aren't necessarily submissive by nature

Safe word: The code word that a submissive can use whenever play becomes too much. A safe word stops all play immediately, and its use is nonnegotiable. A safe word is particularly important in scenes where resistance play is expected; for instance, when a submissive may say "no" as part of the play. Try using "green," "yellow," and "red"—just like a stoplight.

Scene: A session of BDSM play. "Scene" can also be used to refer to the BDSM community as a whole.

Sensation play: A type of BDSM activity that plays with a submissive's sensations. For instance, this may involve hot wax, ice, abrasive materials, or fur. This may or may not escalate into pain play.

Slave: A person who lives the BDSM lifestyle 24/7 and has committed to being under their master's or mistress's control entirely. This is the other role in a TPE.

Soft limits: The boundaries over which a person may cross, if the situation is right. Soft limits are fun to explore, but a person should never be coerced into going beyond what they are comfortable with.

Subdrop: The "low" feeling that a submissive may experience after a particularly intense scene or play session. Although correct aftercare can mitigate these feelings, the "down" state can last for hours or even days.

Submissive (or sub): A person who assumes a more submissive, passive role in a power exchange. Although this is usually sexual, some submissives are service-oriented in that they seek to serve a master or mistress in a practical way without any overt sexual power exchange.

Subspace: The dreamy, euphoric state into which submissives can fall during a particularly intense scene or play session. In subspace, the rest of the world seems to fall away, and the feeling of bliss can last for hours or even days afterward.

Switch: A person who switches between top and bottom roles.

Top: A person who plays a dominant role when required. A top may only play as top for the enjoyment of their master, for instance, and may be more naturally a submissive.

Total power exchange (TPE): A relationship in which one person (the slave) voluntarily and consensually gives another (the master/mistress) total control and authority over them. This is generally a 24/7 agreement and may be open-ended, or may last for a finite time.

Communication

Communication isn't a one-and-done thing; it's a sustained conversation with a partner before, during, and after play. Even when topics feel awkward or uncomfortable, communication is essential for a mutually positive experience and insures that no one gets injured physically or emotionally.

Before You Start

Before you start busting out the rope, you'll need to have a talk with your partner about what you want to go down. Discuss your histories—or lack thereof—with any type of bondage or kinky play, including what worked, and what didn't.

Talk about what you want out of the experience in as much detail as possible.

Be honest and share your deepest fantasies. Do you want to be tied up with your teddy bear and a can of peas? Be brave and say it. Some of your kinks won't overlap, but some will—and it's super-hot when you discover a mutual perviness you can explore.

Talk about your limits.

Hard limits are things that there is no way in hell you're doing—maybe getting peed on or biting. No shame—everyone has stuff they won't do. Accept each other's limits with no judgment. Soft limits are things you might want to explore, but need to tread carefully around and be led through—with the usual option to abort mission at any time.

Agree on a safe word that either of you can use if one of you needs something to stop immediately.

You can use a safe word any time and for any reason. Think of something personal or feel free to be completely basic and use the stoplight system of "green" for "this is good," "yellow" for "this is getting near dangerous territory for me," and "red" for "we need to stop this right now." If a partner is going to be gagged, figure out a non-verbal safe word like hitting a nearby object onto the floor.

Don't forget to include any other issues that might come up. Do you have a trick arm? Claustrophobia? Hatred of the word "moist"? Now's the time to lay it all out.

During

Keep the communicating going throughout your session. Check in with each other regularly, either verbally or non-verbally. Simple questions like "Is this too tight?" or "Does this feel comfortable?" will help ensure that the session is working for both of you. The person being tied up should feel free to ask for any adjustments as you go along. Is your hand getting tingly? Do you need to shift position? Say it. Keep a close eye on each other—are there things that aren't being said that maybe should be? Ask.

If someone uses the safe word, it means you need to stop whatever is happening. But it doesn't necessarily mean the session is over. Check in to see what's happening, talk about whatever issues might have come up, and see how it might be rectified. If you can work through it or fix the problem, you're good to go.

After

Aftercare is a huge part of any bondage experience. With any BDSM scene, you're treading in dangerous territory—that's what makes it so hot—so you need to ensure that everyone emerges from a session both psychologically and physically safe. Aftercare is the time when you both wind down, process the experience, and help each other gently return to regular life.

The first priority of aftercare is attending to any physical effects of a scene. Seek immediate medical attention for any serious injury. Sterilize and bandage any cuts, bruises, or abrasions. Drink water, clean up, and have a cuddle.

After making sure everyone's physically okay, attend to emotional needs. During play, the submissive can get into a state of euphoria called subspace. When it ends, there's a "subdrop" when those happy chemicals flee the scene and the sub can feel sad, vulnerable, and/or exhausted. A good Dom will make their sub feel cared for and nurtured after a session with gentle touch, affirming words, or by fetching a favorite drink. Make sure both partners get the aftercare they need. Let yourselves abandon whatever roles or persona you took on during the scene. Take the time to reflect together on what happened and process whatever came up.

Good aftercare can be as intense and intimate as any sex. Discuss what you want beforehand to make sure you both get what you want

Safety

Good safety practices lead to better bondage play for everyone involved. Make sure you're adhering to the following guidelines before, during, and after your sessions.

Choosing a partner

Finding someone you trust is essential to a safe and positive experience for both of you. You are entering into delicate emotional and physical territory, and you both need to feel completely comfortable with each other. A good partner is open to talking about whatever issues might come up in a session and clearly respects your boundaries. It's easiest if you already have a partner who is interested in exploring bondage, but if you don't, you can get involved with a local fetish community. Websites like FetLife can help you find people with every permutation of kinkiness, but you need to vet anyone thoroughly and in a public place before meeting them in private. If you get even the slightest feeling that someone's not right for you, don't take it further. Never get into any bondage or BDSM scenario with a stranger.

Consent

Consent is affirmative permission given in sound mind. Enthusiastic mutual consent is crucial. Without consent, there can be no play. Badgering or bullying someone into agreeing is not consent. People who are drunk or high can't give consent. Without consent, it's abuse. Consent can be revoked by either of you at any time, for any reason. No exceptions. If someone is not on board with this, stay away.

Safe sex

Know the sexual history of everyone you get involved with. Get tested for sexually transmitted infections beforehand and be open and honest about your status. Don't accept an "I'm clean" from a partner without documentation. Keep a store of condoms, dental dams, and/or latex gloves in reach and use them. Clean and sterilize all toys, sheets, restraints, and surfaces after a session.

Using your equipment safely

You need to be able to get your partner out of any restraint in a matter of seconds. If you're using rope, tape, leather, string, wool, cord, or anything else that can be cut, keep EMT shears nearby. Buy a pair with bright handles so you can find them quickly and keep them right next to you. EMT safety shears are designed to cut without hurting the skin. Avoid using a knife or regular scissors. If you're using handcuffs, keep the key on your regular keychain so it doesn't get lost. Avoid combination locks; it's too easy to forget the code.

If you're using duct tape or anything else that's non-breathable, keep it away from your partner's nose and never wrap it (or anything) around someone's neck. Don't use non-breathable material around the torso either; your partner needs space to breathe.

Make sure the bindings aren't too tight by keeping them loose enough to slide two fingers under them. Check in with your partner regularly to make sure they're comfortable and be alert for signs of poor circulation like discolored skin, tingling sensations, or numbness.

Safety during a session

Don't combine bondage with drugs or excessive booze. A glass of wine beforehand can be okay but anything more than that means impaired judgement which is no bueno.

> Don't tie yourself up without someone else there. And never, ever leave someone alone when they're restrained. EVER. It's super dangerous. Do not do it.

The Equipment

Making sure you have the right equipment on hand will help make for a safer, more comfortable, and all-around better experience for everyone.

Rope

Rope is versatile, easy to use, and it looks innocent if someone stumbles upon it in a drawer.

You can choose from an array of natural and synthetic materials, each with different pros and cons. Natural fibers like jute or hemp hold knots well, but they can feel rough. Cotton is easier on the skin, but isn't as strong as other natural fibers and the knots don't hold as well.

Synthetic ropes are a good choice for beginners. Try soft nylon rope—it's cheap, easy to work with, and is gentle on a sub's skin. Nylon is also easy to clean, holds knots well, and is easy to untie when you've had your way with it.

Touch any rope before you buy it to assess how it will feel against your partner's skin. Avoid polypropylene ropes like the ones for waterskiing (too rough) and climber's rope (too thick).

Whatever type of rope you chose, make sure you have enough on hand. Five feet (1.5 m) of rope is a good minimum. Look for rope that's thinner than ½ inch (1.3 cm). Anything thicker than that will be difficult to maneuver. After you get the rope, you can fix the ends so it doesn't fray. For natural fibers, just tie a knot on each end or wrap them with electrical tape. For nylon, you can melt the ends.

Non-rope options

If you don't have rope on hand or want to DIY it, there are plenty of regular household items you can put into service. You can tie someone up with neckties, long scarves, a belt, or a pair of tights. Duct tape also works, but if you don't love the part where you have to rip it off like a bandage, try specially designed bondage tape which doesn't stick to skin and is reusable. You can also spring for a pair of cuffs. Opt for something with a soft luxe fabric that will be comfortable against the sub's skin. (Metal cop-style cuffs aren't actually a good choice because they'll cut against the sub's wrists.) Don't use any expensive equipment that you'd be hesitant to cut off or ruin in an emergency.

What to put in a bondage kit

Your kit will vary according to what's going down, but here are some ideas for a good starter kit:

- Rope, cuffs, or whatever you'll be using for the bondage
- EMT shears
- A first-aid kit, including bandages, antiseptic wipes, ice packs, and arnica for bruises
- Safe sex items like condoms, dental dams, and latex gloves
- Sex toys like dildos, vibrators, anal plugs, or whatever you're into, plus plenty of lube
- Aftercare comfort items including a soft blanket, water, tissues, and a favorite treat

Bondage Dos and Don'ts

Safety is essential so if the last few pages fell under "too long; did not read," at the very least keep these basic dos and don'ts in mind as you go into any session:

DON'T:

- EVER leave someone in bondage alone.
- Let rope cut into the body.
- Make ties too tight.
- Tie rope, cord, or anything else around the throat.
- Buy anything that you won't be comfortable cutting off someone in an emergency.
- Approach hard limits. Ever.
- Drink or take drugs before playtime.
- Play with a partner who you don't trust 100 percent.
- Ignore someone's discomfort.
- Coerce partners into doing something outside of their comfort zone.

DO:

- Know the health history, sexual and otherwise, of any play partners.
- Always have EMT shears, seatbelt cutters, bolt cutters, and first-aid equipment nearby.
- Check in with your partner throughout a bondage scene.
- Engage in good negotiation and communication before, during, and after a session.
- Approach soft limits with caution.
- Be clean and sanitary.
- Practice safe sex.
- Set a safe word.
- Ensure that bondage takes place in a fun, comfortable, and honest environment.
- Have fun playing, but take safety seriously.

Now that we've covered the essential background information, it's time to show you the ropes.

Let's get knotty.

CHAPTER 1

BASIC KNOTS

Here are some basic knots to get you started. These knots will be your bondage alphabet. Find a willing chair or firm pillow to learn and practice these knots on until you feel confident that you know what you're doing. Then you will be ready to go forth and tie.

New riggers need to learn basic knots before going straight to fancy full-body bondage ties for a couple reasons.

1 - Fumbling over advanced ties will not convey the commanding vibe you're going for.

2 - More importantly, if you don't have the basics down, it can be dangerous. If you place supporting knots in places they shouldn't go, you can injure your sub. Work at the level you can handle and appreciate your own limitations when someone's safety is literally in your hands.

Bula Bula

Ready to start tying? Your first knot is the Bula Bula, the most basic knot for beginners. It is simple, easy to learn, and easy to use. If you don't want to start with someone's actual arm, you can practice on a rolled-up towel.

The Bula Bula is a good knot for starting your ties. It can be tied quickly and efficiently, but it's not recommended for rope bondage suspension.

HOW TO DO IT:

1. Fold your rope in half and wrap the middle part around the wrist or ankle three times. After completing the wraps, cross both ends perpendicularly. Keep the wraps loose; you don't want them too tight at this stage or you won't be able to proceed to the next steps.

2. Tuck the bight end (the loop or bent part) of the rope under the wraps, hook it with your thumb or finger, and pull it through.

3. Make a loop on the other end of the rope with the ends hanging down.

4. Pull the bight end through the loop.

5. Tighten the whole knot and you're done!

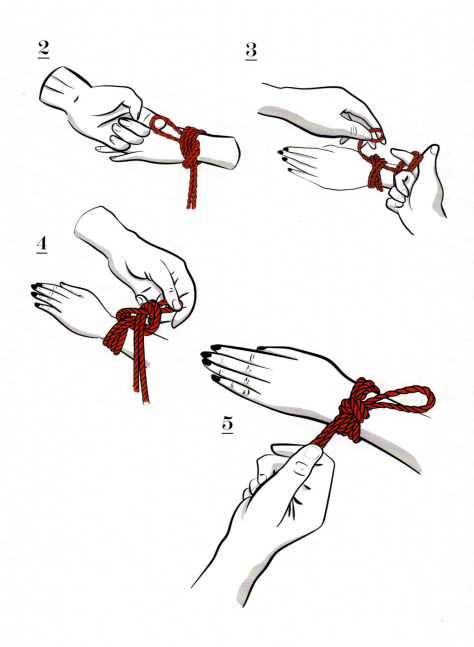

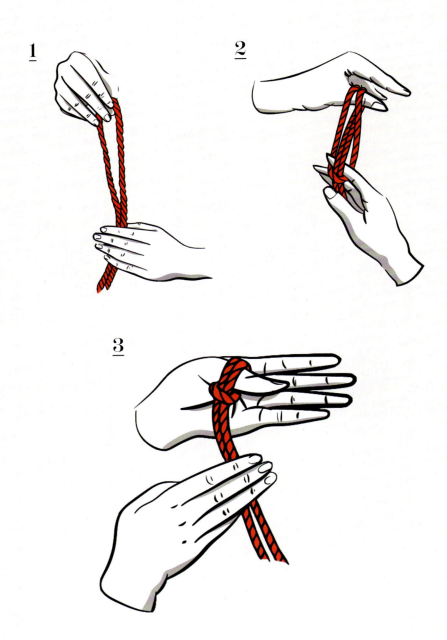

Lark's Head Knot

The Lark's Head Knot (a.k.a. a Cow Hitch) is a gateway knot into more artistic rope bondage. A Hitch Knot is a type of knot used to secure a rope to an object or another rope. It's also a constriction knot, which means that the harder you pull, the tighter it gets. This is a super-versatile knot that can be slipped over the ends of the rope or tied in the middle of a rope when you need a tight knot that won't slide around.

HOW TO DO IT:

1. Create a loop in the middle of the rope. The loop is called the bight end.
2. Wrap it around your thumb and pull the long end through.
3. Tighten the knot and you're done!

Munter Hitch

This knot is used mostly for decorative crossovers and changes of direction in rope bondage. It makes your rope bondage look more polished when crossing rope than if you just loop it around. Make sure you keep steady pressure on the knot while tying it or else it falls apart.

HOW TO DO IT:

1. Place the bight end of the first rope perpendicularly over a second piece of rope that you want to tie on to.
2. Bring the bight end of the first rope under the second rope.
3. Next, bring it across and over the end of the same piece of rope you're tying.
4. Cross back under the second rope. That's it! Carry on with the rest of your bondage.

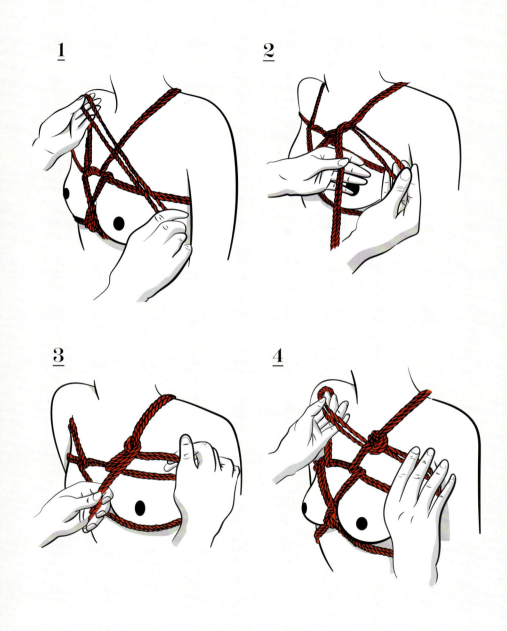

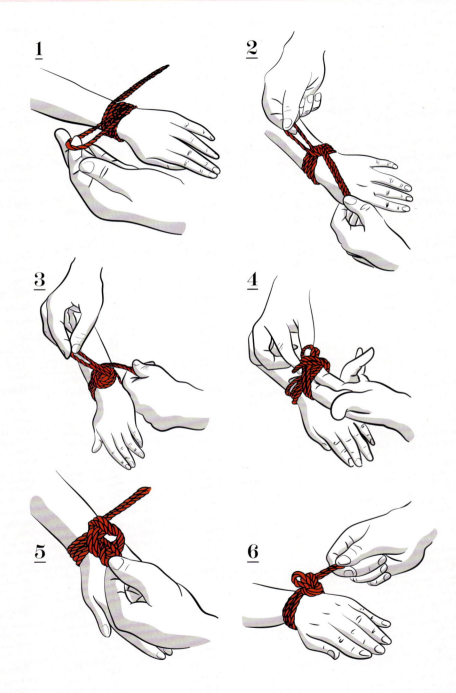

Sommerville Bowline

This unidirectional knot is great for starting intermediate ties. Once it's snug, you should have a rope "cuff" that won't constrict the wrist. The bonus of this knot is that it holds in all directions and is easy to untie.

HOW TO DO IT:

1. Grasp the length of rope in the middle, then wrap it around your partner's wrist three times. It doesn't have to be tight—in fact, a little slack is best.

2. After you have done the three wraps, take the ends and cross them perpendicularly.

3. Wrap the long end under and around the back of the bight.

4. Push two fingers through the large loop you just made and under all the wraps around the wrist.

5. Bend the short end backward and grasp it with the fingers you just pushed through the loop, then pull that end back through the loop.

6. Pull to tighten the whole knot evenly. You're done!

BASIC KNOTS

Joining Rope

This is a tidy-looking technique for adding more rope when you get to the end of a rope. It's also good for adding rope when you (inevitably) get to a point where the ends of your rope aren't the same length. The end that's too long won't have any tension and there will be slack. Creating a habit of knotting the end of your ropes makes this an easy fix.

HOW TO DO IT:

1. Make a knot on each end of the rope.
2. Take the longer end and fold it back on itself so that the newly created loop end is the same length as the knot end.
3. Slip a Lark's Head (page 23) around the two ends and tighten.

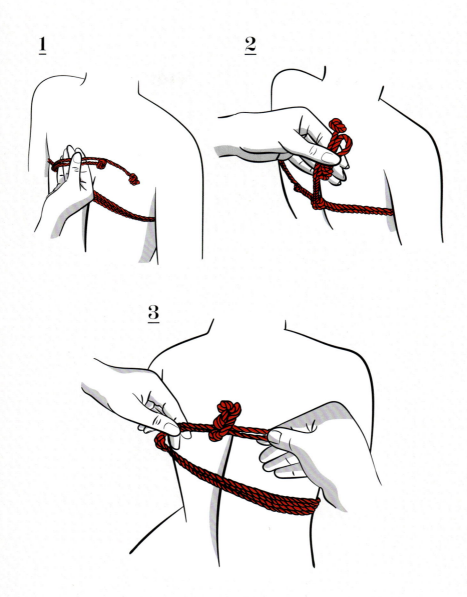

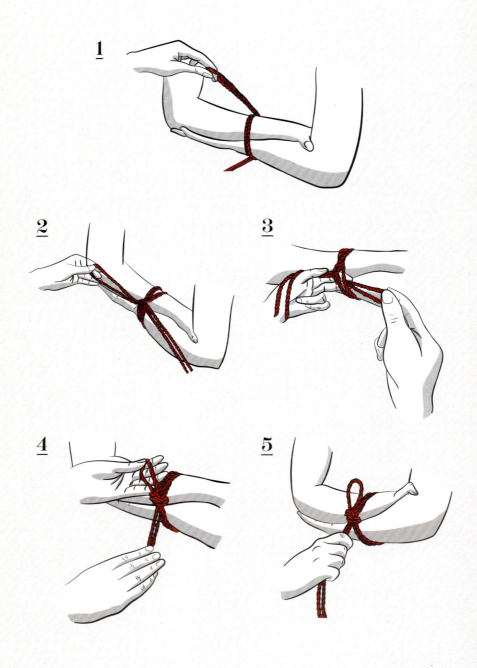

Wrists Behind

Tying someone's wrist behind them can make them feel off balance. To make your partner feel safer, have them sit on a bed or chair while you're binding them. After they're bound, they won't have use of their arms, so make sure they don't fall down.

HOW TO DO IT:

1. Have your partner fold their arms behind their back with one forearm resting on top of the other. Wrap the bight end or your rope around both of their wrists.

2. Cross the bight end perpendicularly so that each end is following the direction ovvf each forearm.

3. Take the loop end and tuck it through the opening between where the arms are folded together and gently but firmly tighten.

4. Finish by topping it off with an Overhand Knot.

5. Enjoy!

BASIC KNOTS

Two-Column Tie

This can be used for binding together any "two columns," like two legs, an arm and a bedpost, or, as in this example, two wrists.

HOW TO DO IT:

1. Have your partner bring their arms together in front of them with about an inch (3 cm) of space between them. Hold the bight end of your rope and wrap it around their wrists a few times.

2. Cross the ends over each other and change direction so the bight is pointing toward your partner.

3. Drop the loop end between the wrists and wrap under and back up between the arms.

4. Tie an Overhand Knot (it doesn't have to be fancy).

5. Add another Overhand Knot on top of that.

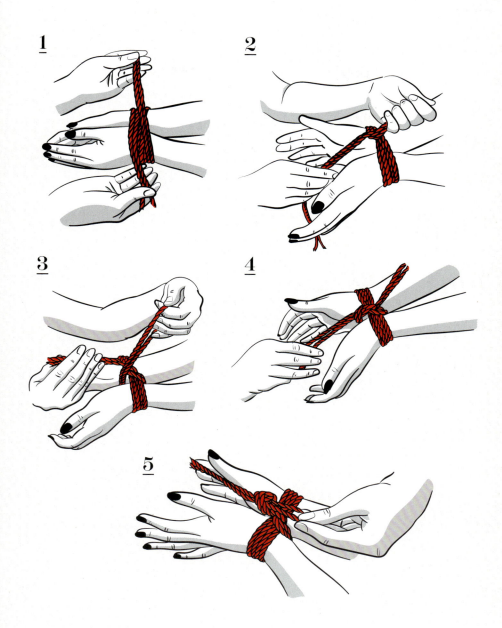

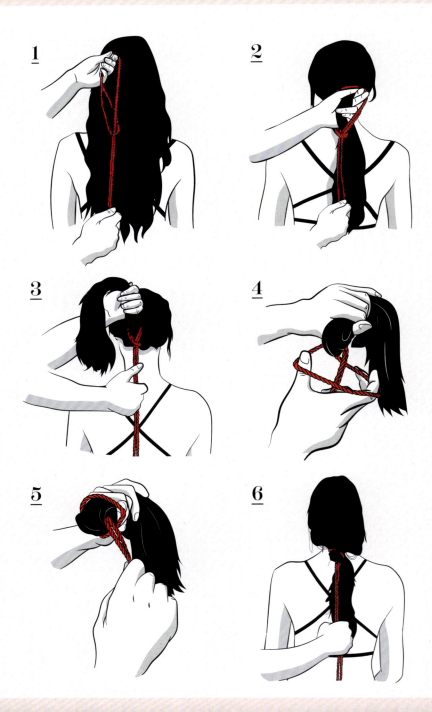

Basic Hair Tie

Arms, legs, and torsos are the basic parts to bind, but you can open a whole new avenue of play with hair tying. You can use a hair tie to hold someone with long hair in place, lead them around, or position them how you want. For the best results, use a long length of rope or thick yarn. Choose something with loose fibers so it will grab onto their hair better. Add a spritz of hairspray to help the rope or yarn grab better.

HOW TO DO IT:

1. Use a hair elastic to put your partner's hair into a ponytail. Use about 16 inches (41 cm) of rope or thick yarn and double it over to 8 inches (20 cm). Make a loop in the middle and pull the ends loosely through in a Lark's Head Knot (page 23).

2. Pull the ponytail all the way through the Lark's Head Knot.

3. Push the Lark's Head up over the hair elastic at the base of the ponytail.

4. Fold the ponytail in half upward and pull the loop open.

5. Push the loop up and over the now doubled ponytail. The main line of the rope should be through the middle of the folded ponytail.

6. Pull it steadily to tighten until you have a snug hold. Take care not to tug any stray hairs.

BASIC KNOTS

Crossed Wrists Tie

This is similar to the Wrist Tie but uses a rope between the wrists so you can keep your partner's wrists crossed. It's a simple and versatile tie that is reasonably comfortable for the person being bound. It also works well for binding ankles.

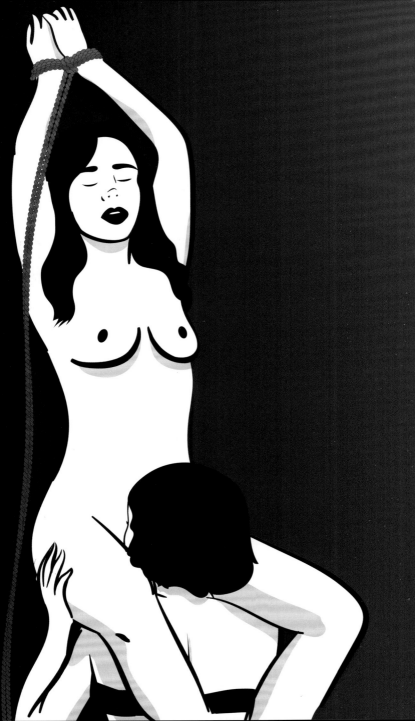

HOW TO DO IT:

1. Fold the rope in half then wrap it around your partner's wrists, making sure the rope is flat with no twists. Cross the rope at the base of the thumb.

2. Wrap the bight end between the wrists.

3. Bring the bight end under and around.

4. Tie it to the free end of the rope on the underside of the arms.

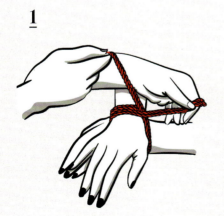

<u>1</u>

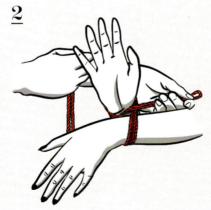

<u>2</u>

38 THE BONDAGE PLAYBOOK

3

4

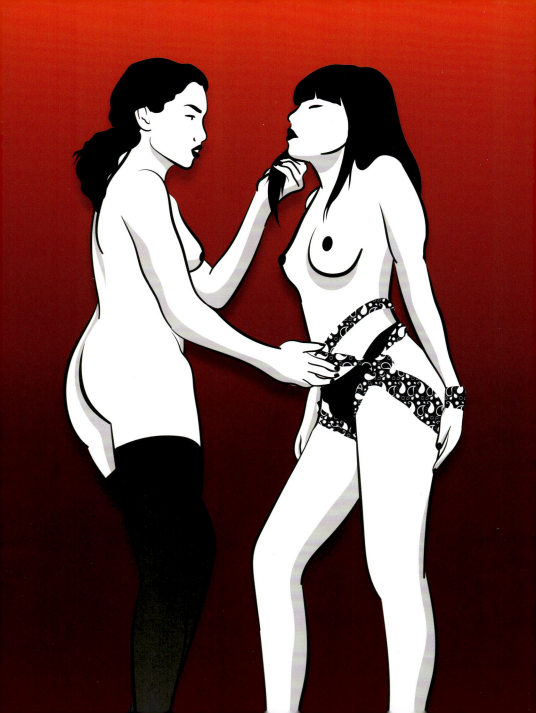

DIY Necktie Sex Harness

If you don't have any rope, you can DIY any of the positions in this book with neckties or long scarves. Here's a way to use neckties to create a spontaneous hip harness to guide your partner.

HOW TO DO IT:

1. Stand behind your partner and wrap the tie around their waist.

2. Make a simple knot over one hip.

3. Wrap the back end of the tie up between the legs and the front end down between the legs to the back, making sure the tie lies flat, not twisted.

4. Bring both ends up and retie a new knot over top of the original one.

5. Repeat with another tie on the other side, making the knots comfortable but not loose.

6. Tuck both ends in and you're ready to go!

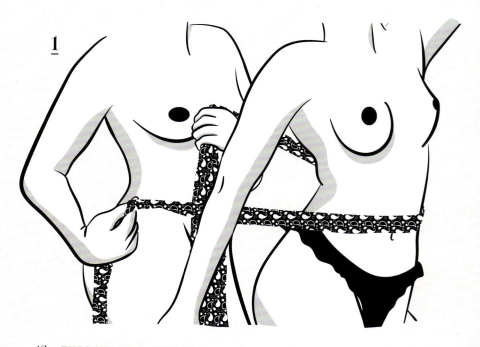

1

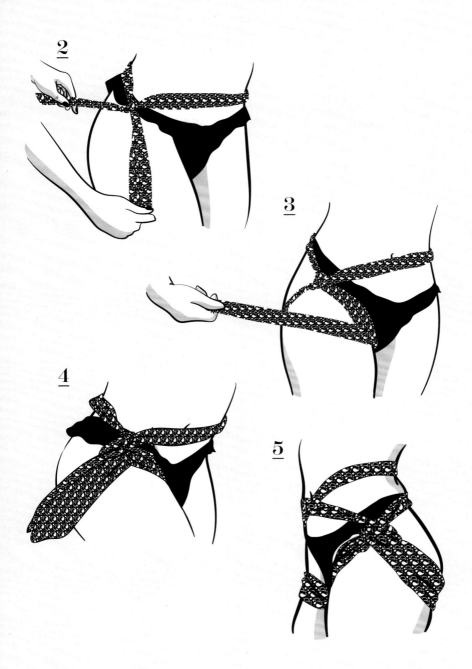

·CHAPTER·
2

THE TIES

Once you've mastered some basic knots, you can take them a little further with more ornate ties. This section has ties to highlight or bind specific body parts, ties to bind your partner into particular positions, and more intricate ties that do the job while looking a bit showier.

Beginner Hair Tie with Braid

This tie is more secure than the tie we learned in chapter 1 because the rope is wound all the way through your bunny's hair. It's easy to learn because it uses a basic braid, plus... it just looks cool.

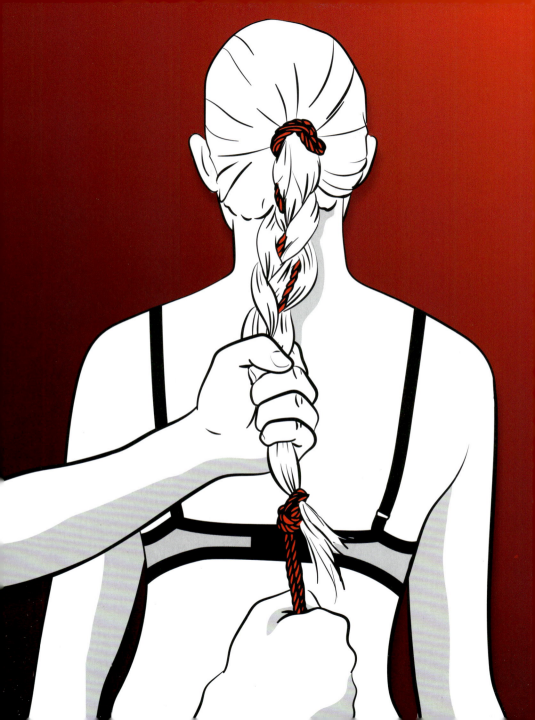

HOW TO DO IT:

1. Use a hair elastic to put your partner's hair into a ponytail. Take the middle of the rope and tie an Overhand Knot around the base of the ponytail.

2. Take the loop part and tuck it down through the hair above the base of the ponytail, against your partner's head.

3. Lift up the ponytail and pull it all the way through, leaving about an inch and a half (4 cm) of loop below the hair.

4. Feed the free end of the rope through the loop and pull it to make it snug. This will be your base to begin braiding.

5. Gather the hair into three sections, putting the two pieces of rope into two of the sections. Braid by taking the middle section and crossing it over the right section, then taking the newly created middle section and crossing it over the left. Repeat to continue.

6. Braid all the way to the end, then form a large loop and pull it through. Tighten at the bottom and you're done!

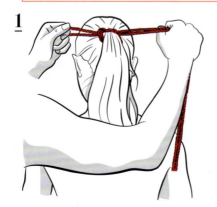
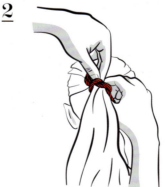

48   THE BONDAGE PLAYBOOK

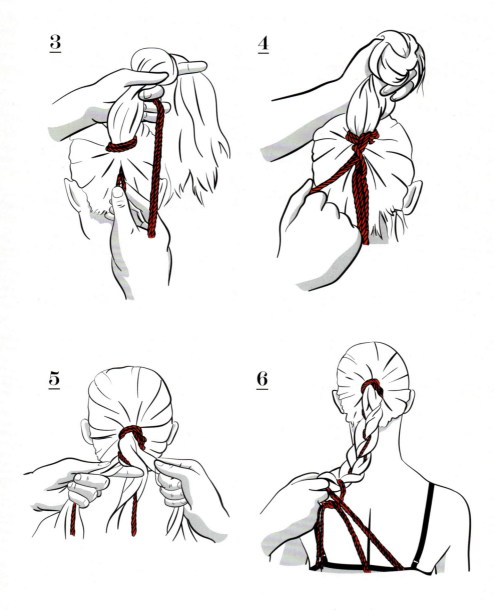

Advanced Hair Tie

This hair tie is as sturdy as the previous hair tie, but it's got a fetishy look you could wear for a night out at a kink party.

HOW TO DO IT:

1. Use a hair elastic to put your partner's hair into a ponytail. Fold a rope in half and bring the bight end up from the bottom, sliding it behind the hair elastic and forming a loop above the hair tie.

2. Bring the two ends of the long rope up over the hair. Feed them through the loop to form a secure base.

3. Make a loop around the ponytail with the free end on the inside of the loop.

4. Pull the loop tight.

5. Move an inch or two (3 to 5 cm) down and repeat step 3 until you reach the end. Finish with an Overhand Knot on the last turn in the rope.

6. Tighten securely and you're done!

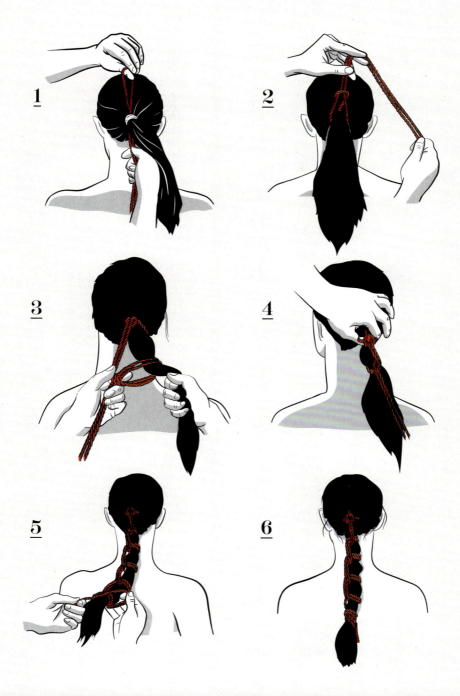

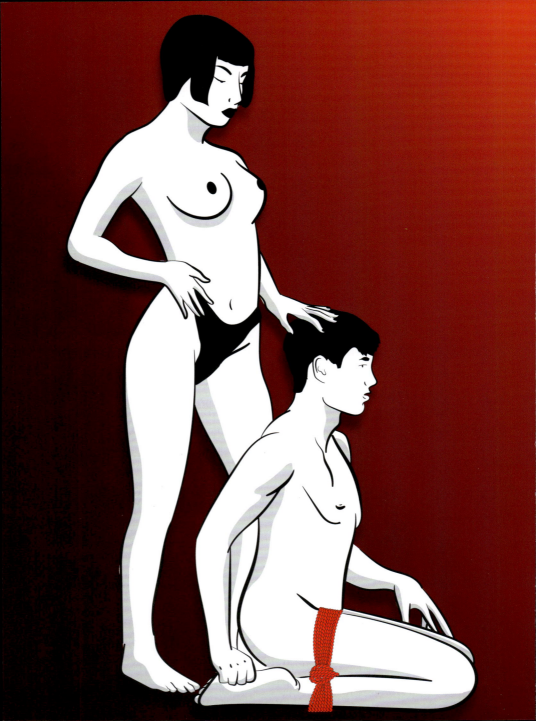

Kneeling Two-Column Leg Tie

Use a Two-Column Tie to bind your partner's legs together and keep them in place. Having a sub kneel before you is a power move, and this is the easiest tie to get them there. This type of bondage has a wide band across the legs so it's more comfortable for the person being tied.

HOW TO DO IT:

1. Have your partner kneel and make three wraps around their leg. Keep the wraps up near the thigh.

2. Finish the wrapping when you have about 14 inches (36 cm) left of the loop end then cross it perpendicularly with the free end.

3. Take the free end, tuck it down, and wrap it around the wraps on the other side.

4. Pull it up again and cinch it tight.

5. Push the loop over the final free end and cinch it down a second time, as in a Bula Bula Knot (page 20).

6. Tuck all your ends in and you're ready to go.

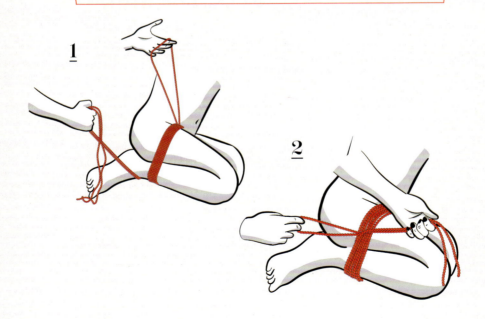

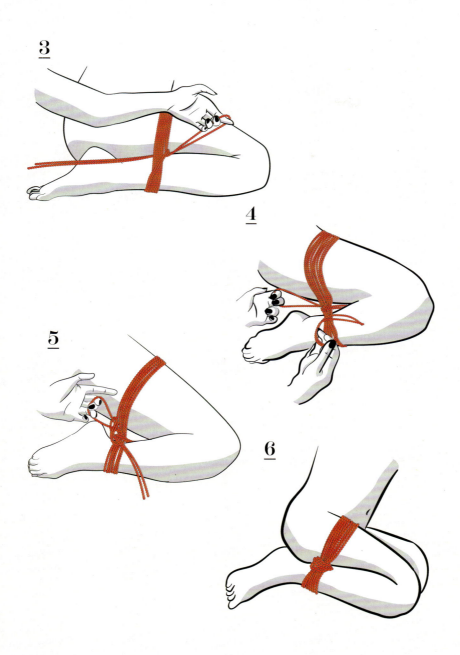

The Arm Binder

A simple arm binder adds a forceful vibe to your play and keeps your partner in place—literally and figuratively. The positioning for this one won't work for everyone's body, which is fine. If they want to give it a go, it can help if they bend forward. If it's not working, don't push it. Stay in communication with your partner, only taking them as far as they want to go. It should not be painful for them.

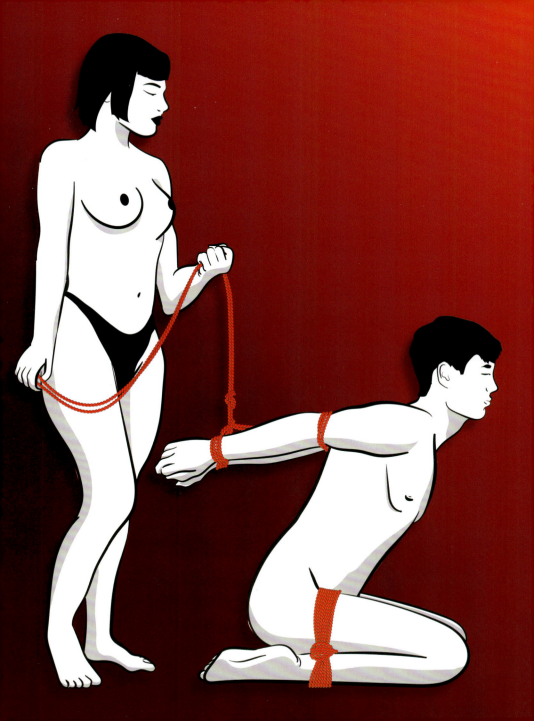

HOW TO DO IT:

1. Have your partner place their arms together behind their back. Tie a basic Two-Column Tie (page 32) around their wrists.

2. Bring the rope up vertically and wrap it around your partner's upper arms, above their elbows. Make sure you have enough tension so the rope won't slip. Your partner can help keep it in place by pushing their arms against the rope as you're wrapping them.

3. After the wraps are on, pass the rope around the middle, as in the Kneeling Tie (page 53). Pick up the wraps on the other side, gently pull the arms together at the elbow, and cinch it down.

4. Take the rope and come over the left shoulder. Instead of crossing the chest, drop the rope down and through the left armpit and bring it across the back.

5. Come across the back, up through the right armpit, over the right shoulder, and then back to the cinch where the elbows trapped.

6. Finish by tying the ends into a festive bow.

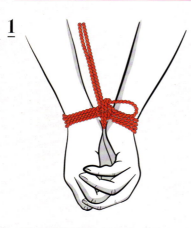

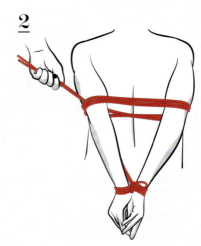

58   THE BONDAGE PLAYBOOK

3

4

5

6

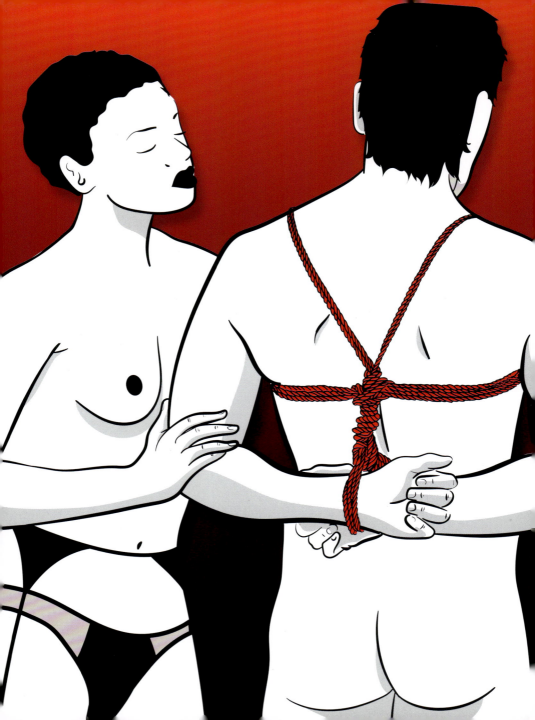

The Broad Chest Harness

This intermediate chest tie accentuates your partner's broad chest while keeping their hands bound behind them. All you need is one length of rope.

HOW TO DO IT:

1. Bind your partner's wrist using the Wrists Behind Tie (page 31). Take the rope over the right shoulder, then down through the right armpit to the back and under the rope.

2. Take the rope across the back, up through the left armpit and over the left shoulder, then back to the center.

3. Wrap the rope around the center point where the ropes meet.

4. Take the rope through the right armpit again, across the chest, and pull it through the left shoulder rope.

5. Come back and under the right shoulder rope.

6. Form a quick Munter Hitch (page 24) in the center of the chest, then go across the chest and through the left armpit to your partner's back to tie it off.

1

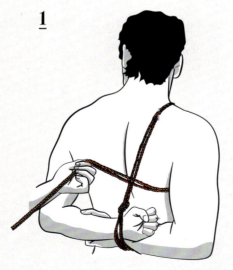

2

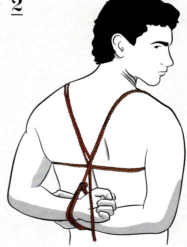

62 THE BONDAGE PLAYBOOK

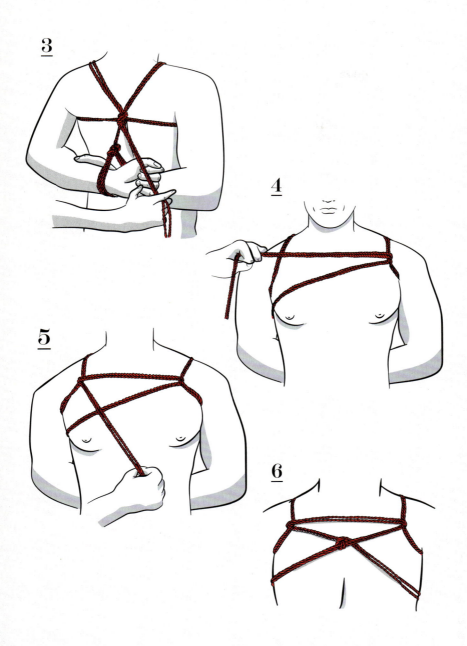

Basic Futo

This is a basic version of a Futo Tie (a Western shorting of Futomoto, a Japanese bondage technique of binding the ankles to the thigh). It is more complicated and ornate than the Two-Column Tie (page 53) but it's more comfortable for your partner and looks more impressive. You'll start with one side, then do the other.

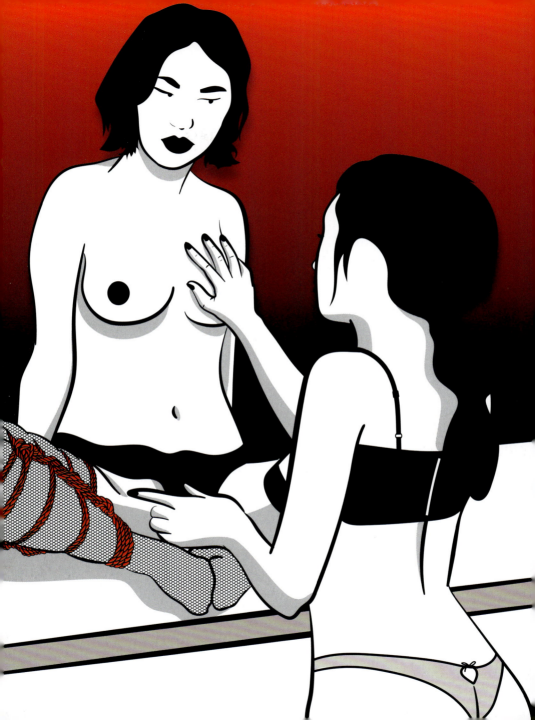

HOW TO DO IT:

1. Start with a simple Bula Bula (page 20) or Sommerville Bowline (page 27) around the ankle.

2. Have your partner sit, bending their leg tight to their body. Start high on their thigh near their hip joint and wrap the rope from the bottom upward, keeping their lower leg pushed against their thigh.

3. Make four wraps, then when you come around the top, bring a final half wrap around to catch the top horizontal wrap.

4. Work your way downward away from the knee, making a simple overhand wrap around each horizontal wrap as you go.

5. Once you've wrapped the rope around the final horizontal wrap, tuck it under that wrap and pull it through to the other side. Have your partner bend their leg forward so you can repeat the process on the outside of the leg, this time working your way upward toward the knee.

6. If you have a lot of rope left once you reach the top of the knee on the outside of the leg, retrace your steps, building a new layer over the top of what you just made, coming back up the inside, wrapping in a twisting motion around all the verticals to keep the rope from getting tangled during the rest of your session. Tie your rope off and you're done!

1
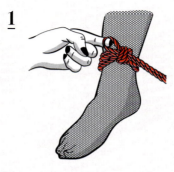

2
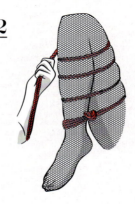

THE BONDAGE PLAYBOOK

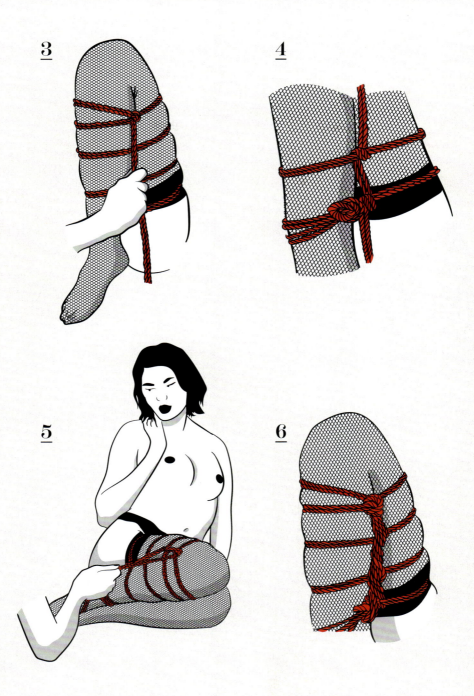

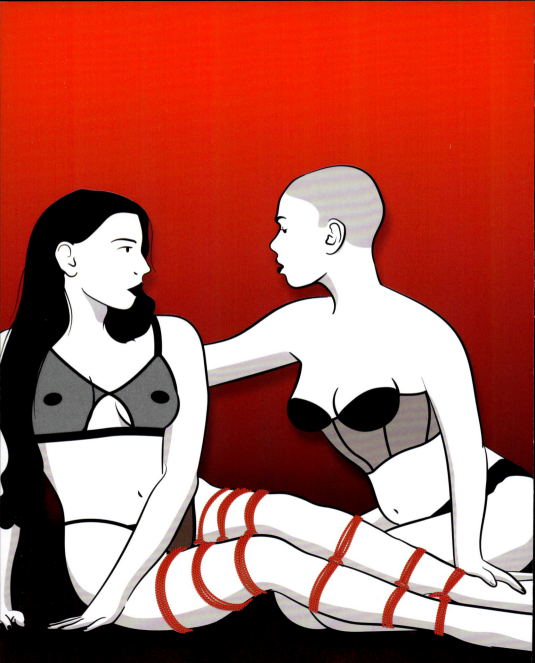

Ladder Tie

A leg binding is great for a partner who likes to feel helpless and totally bound. Have them lie down for this tie so they don't fall over. If you have enough rope and a willing partner, you can continue the tie all the way up the body.

HOW TO DO IT:

1. Tie a Two-Column Tie (page 32) around your partner's ankles.

2. Bring the rope to the back of their legs and wrap it twice around the shins.

3. Tuck the rope up and over the wraps on the other side of the vertical rope.

4. Keep the tension on the rope and bring it between the leg and up over the shin wraps.

5. Come back through and make a wrap around the vertical rope again.

6. Repeat this series of wraps all the way up the body, making wraps every 10 inches (25 cm). Tie just below and above the knees—not right on the joint. Tie off and you're done!

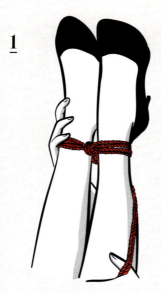

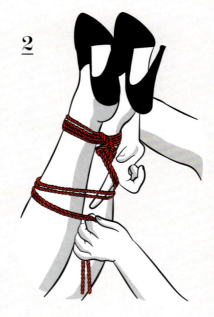

70   THE BONDAGE PLAYBOOK

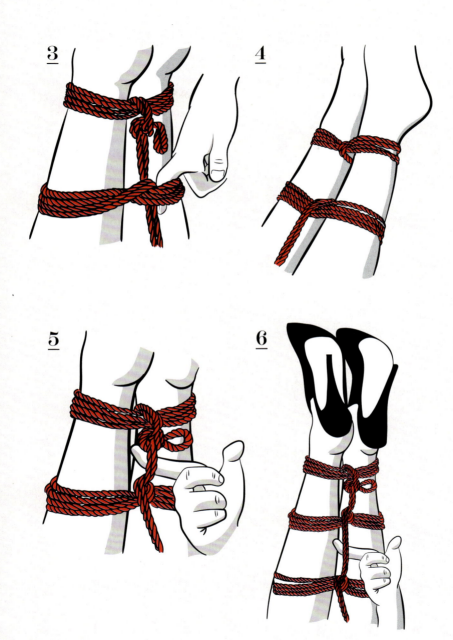

Asymmetric Broad Chest Tie

This asymmetrical tie looks different on both sides. It's a strong tie that you can use over clothes before pulling them off. If you want to add some extra dominance, bend your partner over and put your knee on their back to hold them in place while you finish the ties in the back.

All the main knots for this tie are in the back so make sure you enjoy the view from behind!

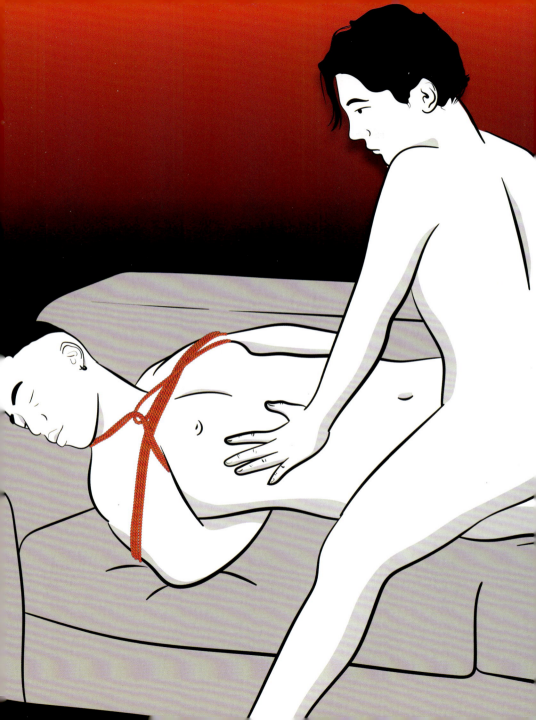

HOW TO DO IT:

1. Tie your partner's hand behind them using a Two-Column Tie (pages 32), then bring the rope up and wrap it to the right around their chest and shoulder, above the nipple line.

2. Once you have two wraps around the chest, bring the rope between their right arm and chest and up over their right shoulder. Then pull the rope down under their left armpit and across the front of the chest.

3. Tuck the rope under the piece going over the right shoulder and double back the way you came—across the chest and back under the left armpit.

4. Use a finger to pull up the lower wrap on the back.

5. Tuck the rope under the lower wrap, cinch it tight, then finish with a knot in the back.

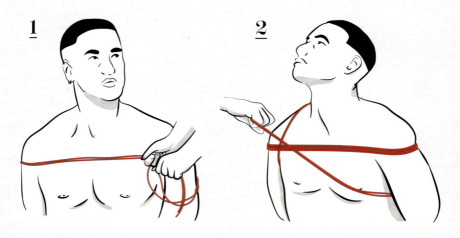

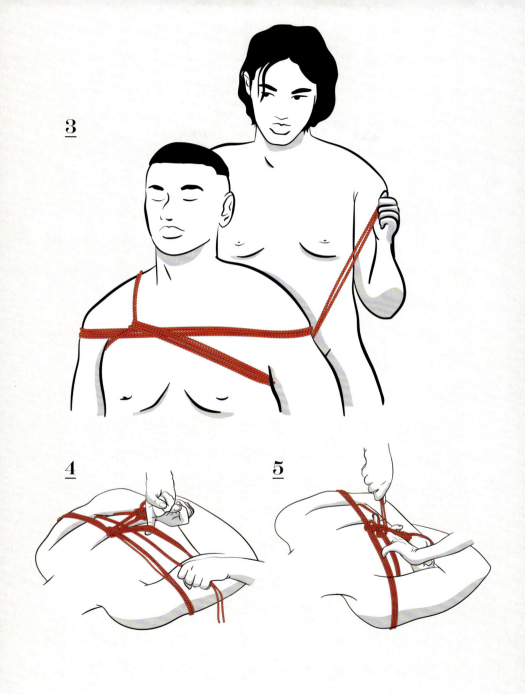

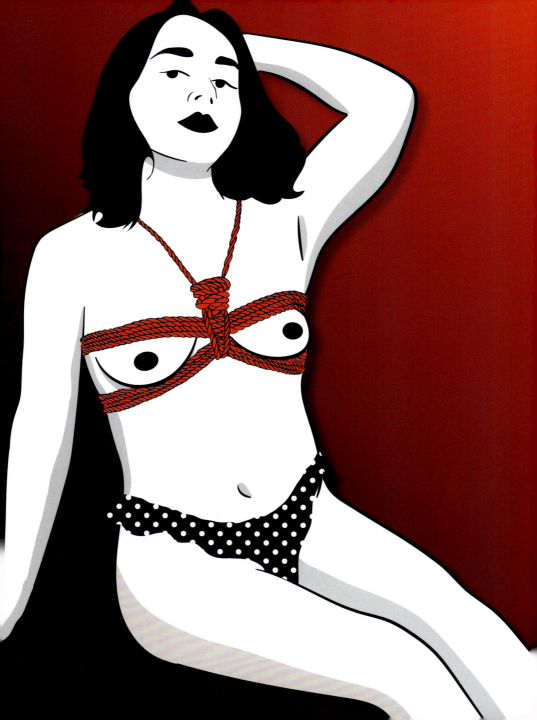

Self-Serve Chest Tie

No one says you need a partner to tie you up! You can bind yourself to highlight a body part or wrap yourself up for a partner. That being said, no one should ever do any type of bondage alone, so you need to have someone with you, even if their hands never touch your rope. And, as with all bondage, keep a pair of safety shears nearby for a quick release.

HOW TO DO IT:

1. Start with a simple loop around your chest, underneath the breasts.
2. Bring the rope through the loop and reverse around the way you came.
3. Find the original loop you created when you passed the rope around the body. Pull that loop open a little and pass the rope back through it.
4. Take the rope straight up between the breasts, holding it in place while you change direction and make a wrap around the chest again, this time above the breasts. Pass the rope under the vertical rope in the center of the chest. Keep the tension in the rope so it doesn't slip down.
5. Reverse the rope as you did before, wrapping it back above your breasts and feeding the rope back through the loop.
6. You can get creative with the finish. You can make a pair of diagonal passes with the rope, then pass the rope around to the back of the body to tie off. Or you can wrap the rope around the back of your neck so it looks like a bra. Or you can bring the rope back under the bottom wraps and tie it to the top wraps. Up to you.

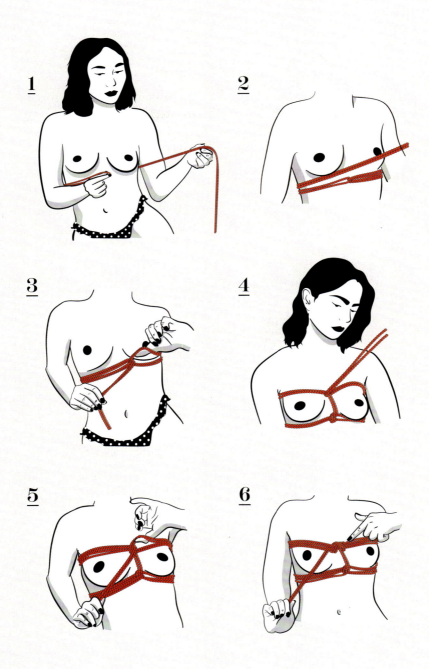

CHAPTER 3
Taking It Further

Now that you've mastered the basic knots and learned to fancy them up a bit, this section will show you how to take it deeper. These knots will help to expand on what you've practiced so you can bind body parts more effectively, combine different types of knots to form new or more elaborate bondage set ups, and extend your ties into harnesses or full-body creations.

Finger Tie

Tying up your partner's fingers removes their ability to touch you or themselves. This can encourage them to use their mouth or feet to touch you or can be a way to restrict their hands as part of a Dom/sub scenario. We recommend using a man-made fiber like acrylic yarn for the fingers. It's thin enough that it will slide easily through the fingers without constricting them, plus it's inexpensive. Make the yarn snug but not so tight that it cuts off their circulation. When you're done, just cut it off and throw it away.

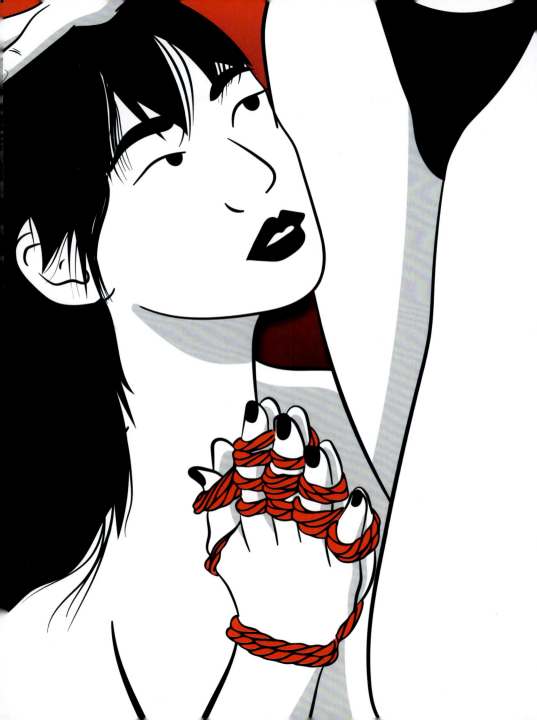

HOW TO DO IT:

1. Wrap a Lark's Head Knot (page 23) around your partner's wrist and then come back through the middle, as in a Two-Column Tie (page 32).

2. Separate the ends and bring each one around under the thumbs.

3. Have your partner spread their fingers, then weave the string between them, wrapping around each one, and binding their hands together.

4. When you get to the end, cross the string around the pinkies and adjust the tension as needed.

5. Weave your way back to the thumbs, going back the way you came, once again wrapping each finger as you go.

6. Tie back between the thumbs or the wrists.

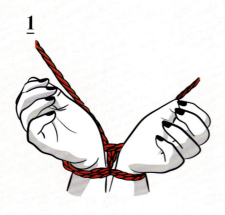

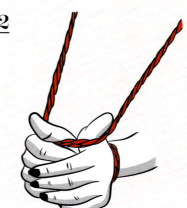

THE BONDAGE PLAYBOOK

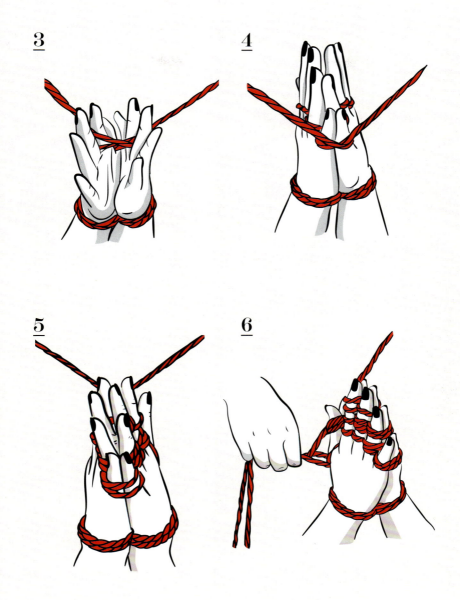

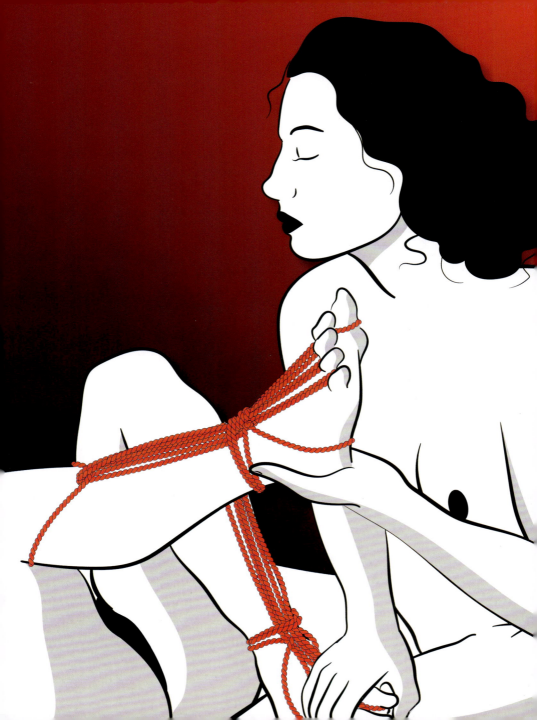

Toe Tie

Toe Ties work well for playing with edging and orgasm denial because—fun fact!—people tend to point or flex their toes when they have an orgasm. If you notice your partner is a flexer or pointer, you can tie their feet and toes the opposite way to make it incredibly hard for them to orgasm without you releasing them. If they can stand it, make them beg for it.

HOW TO DO IT:

1. Make a tie under the knee, above the calf, then make a loop in the front. (The bulge of the calf will hold this loop in place.) Keep it loose enough so there's space for a few fingers under it. Bring the yarn down and wrap it around the big toe, then return to the calf loop.

2. Repeat this step, bringing the yarn down to wrap around the second, then third toe.

3. Continue until you get to the fourth toe. (We don't normally tie the pinkie.)

4. Bring the yarn up to make a big wrap around the ankle, pulling the strands into one bundle, then tying it off. Repeat this with the other foot if desired!

<u>1</u>

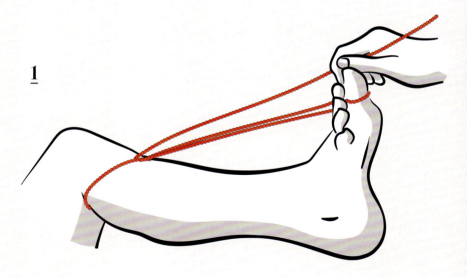

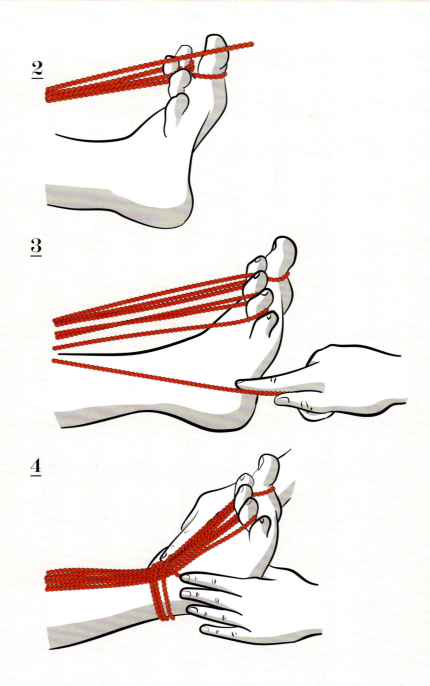

Simple Chest Harness

This Simple Chest Harness works well on its own to highlight your partner's chest or as a foundation for creating something more complex. (It works particularly well if the person being tied has breasts, as it provides support and makes them stand up a little prouder!) If you have extra rope when you make the finishing tie, you can use it to bind your partner's wrists as well.

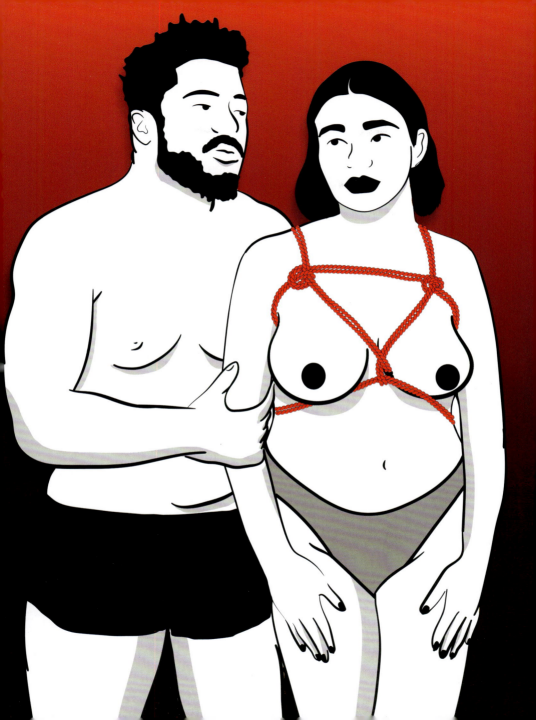

HOW TO DO IT:

1. Fold the rope in half to create a bight (loop). Wrap the rope around the torso, just under the breasts, and pull the ends through the bight in the center of the back.

2. Bring the rope up and over the shoulder and down to the middle. Cross over and under the rope just under the breasts in the center of the torso, then go back up again over the opposite shoulder.

3. Pull the rope over the shoulder and bring it up and under the horizontal wrap. Pull it up between the wrap and the base of the left shoulder rope and make a simple knot to hold it secure.

4. Come around the front, under the arm, and pull the rope from under the shoulder outward. Form a Munter Hitch (page 24) here.

5. Bring the rope across the chest and tie another Munter's Hitch on the shoulder rope on the other side.

6. Bring the rope around to your partner's back to tie it off. If you have extra rope, you can tie it around their wrists.

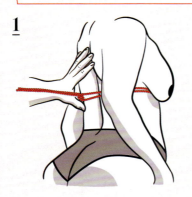

1

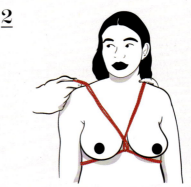

2

92   THE BONDAGE PLAYBOOK

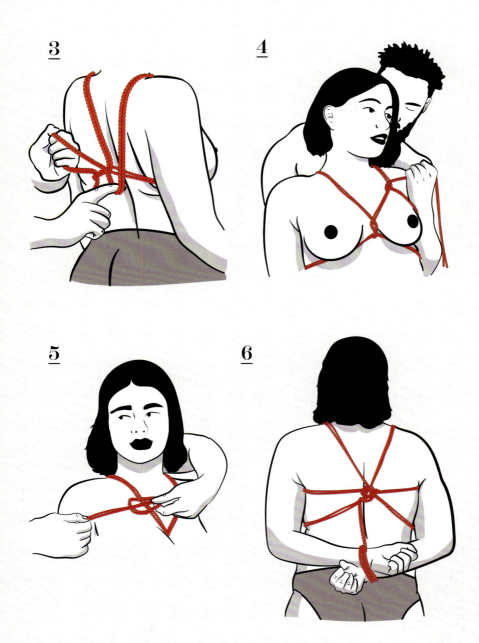

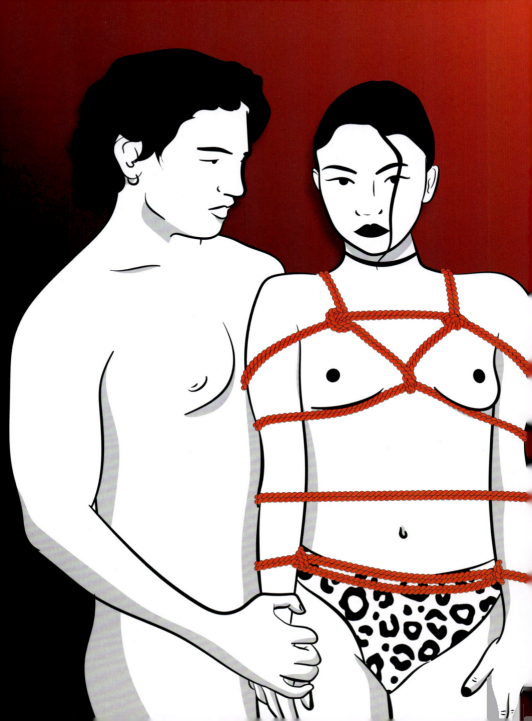

Simple Chest Harness with Wrist Capture

This is a variation on the Simple Chest Harness (page 90) that includes wrist binding. But instead of binding your partner's wrists behind their back, you'll bind their wrists so they're pinned to their sides.

Make sure you have enough rope to add the wrist capture to this harness.

HOW TO DO IT:

1. Start with the Simple Chest Harness (page 90), but have your partner relax their arms at their sides so they're captured there as you create the harness. When the harness is complete, bring the ends of the rope down and create a loop around their body, trapping the arms just above the wrists.

2. Bring the rope around the one running down the middle of your partner's back.

3. Bring the rope to a wrist and feed it on the inside of their wrist.

4. Bring the rope up and over the rope that captures the wrist, pulling it back through the way you just came, so that you're cinching the wrists snugly. Go back around and do the other wrist.

5. Come back around the rope, down the spine, and make a loop around the rope.

6. Knot it all off in the back, tying neatly.

1
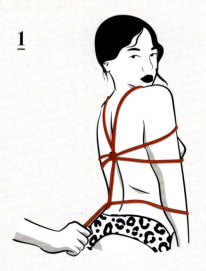

2
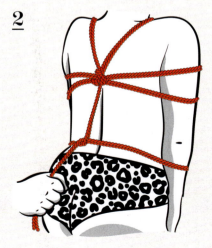

96 THE BONDAGE PLAYBOOK

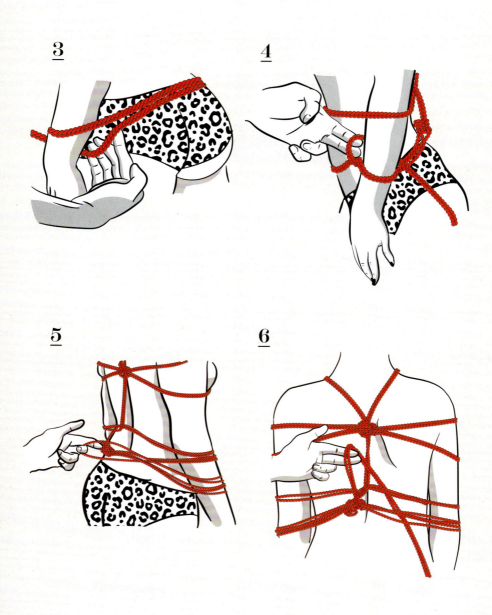

Elevated Chest Harness

Here's a slightly more complex—but still doable!—chest harness. Use it to accentuate a wide chest or a great pair of boobs. You can also use it as a handle to lead your partner around or hold them in place.

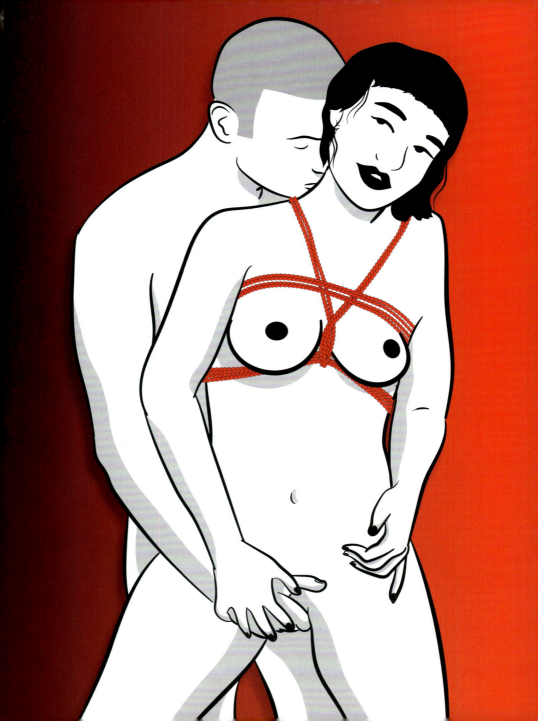

HOW TO DO IT:

1. Make a Lark's Head Knot (page 23) around your partner's rib cage.

2. Wrap the rope twice around your partner's ribs, right below their breasts.

3. Bring the rope up and make two wraps above the breasts.

4. Pull the free end through the loops you made earlier at the back.

5. Take the rope over the shoulder and down between the breasts, wrap it around the lower wraps, and then give it an extra twist as you come back up over the right shoulder.

6. Tie the rope off at their back. For extra finesse, you can use the leftover rope to weave it back and forth between the shoulder ropes.

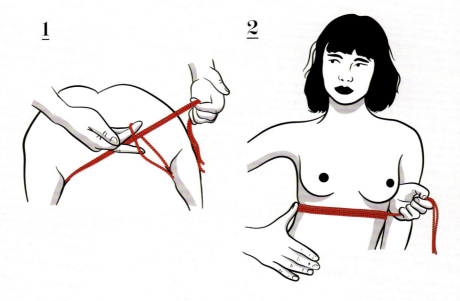

100   THE BONDAGE PLAYBOOK

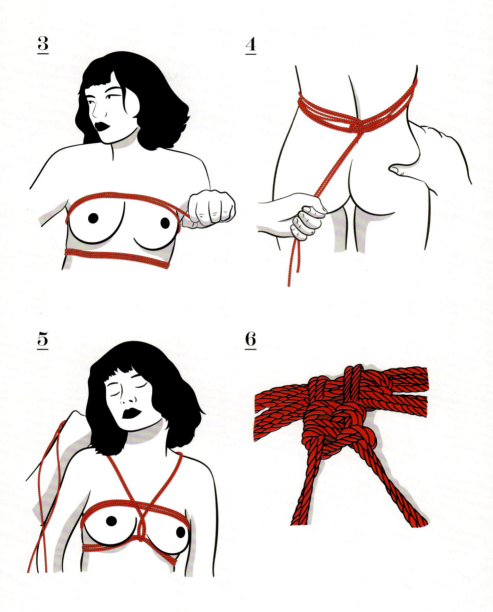

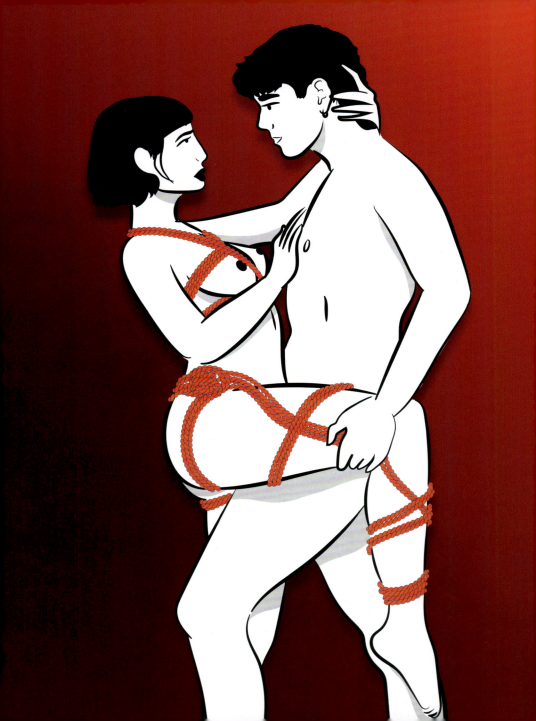

Simple Hip Harness and Leg Weave

Use the Simple Hip Harness and Leg Weave as a stand-alone design or combine it with the Elevated Chest Harness (page 98) for a more complex full-body harness. It makes a great handle for guiding your partner into place and keeping them there. Try it with sex from behind, either penetrative or with a mouth or toy.

HOW TO DO IT:

1. Start with the Elevated Chest Harness (page 98). Have your partner stand with their hands against a wall and tie a Lark's Head Knot (page 23) around their waist.

2. Wrap around the waist twice and then make a Half Hitch on the hip. (Reminder: A Hitch Knot is type of knot used to secure a rope to an object or another rope.)

3. Bring the rope across the front of your partner's thigh, down between their legs, and up the crease where the hip and bum meet the leg, all the way up to the original hitch on the side. Then go over the wrap you just made, under the waist wraps, over the hitch, and under the bottom wrap.

4. Repeat, following the same path, making the opposite weave right beside the line you are following.

5. Once you get the waist harness looking the way you want, you can use another length of rope and start winding down and around the thigh and leg. Remember to weave the opposite way as you trace back through.

6. Tie the rope off and enjoy!

1

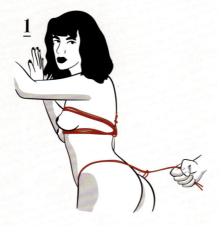

2

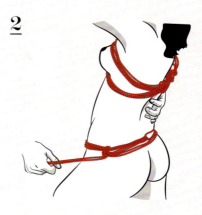

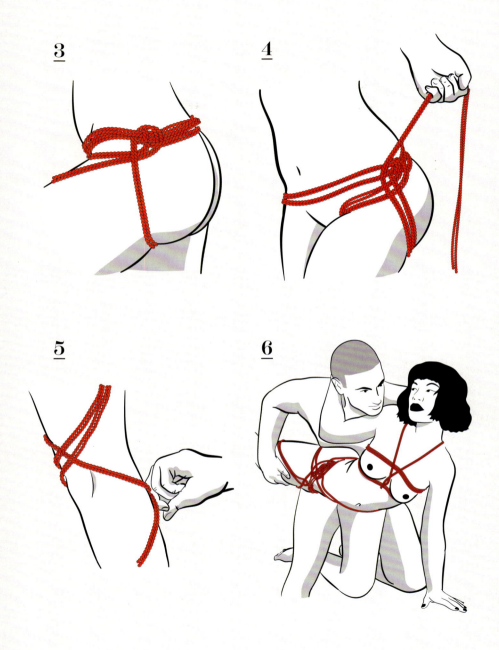

Beginner Sex Harness Hip Tie

This is the bondage equivalent to crotchless panties. It offers easy access to butt and groin, plus you can hold onto it to put your partner exactly where you want them—just pull them into place. It uses a weaving technique so there are minimal knots to tie.

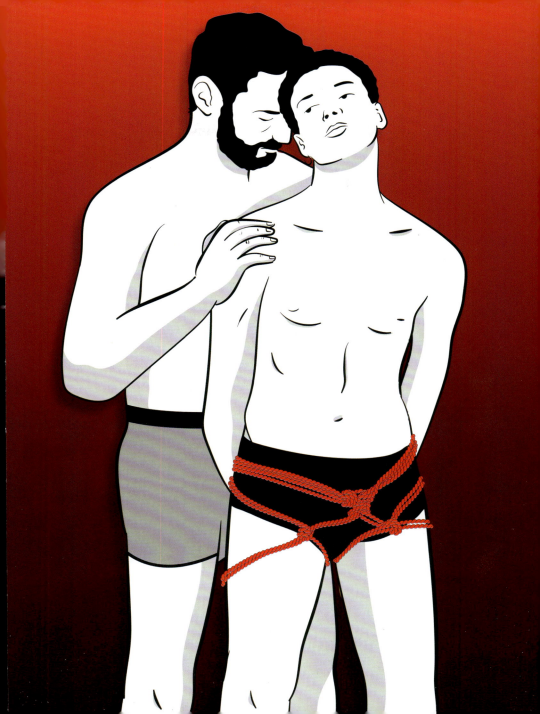

HOW TO DO IT:

1. Start with a simple hip wrap going twice around the body and finishing with a Bula Bula (page 20) or a Sommerville Bowline (page 27) in the front of your partner's body, just above their crotch.

2. Bring the rope over the thigh, under the bum, and up between the legs.

3. Connect to the thigh rope with a Munter Hitch (page 24) and pull through.

4. Bring that rope around the back and make a quick Hitch Knot to keep the rope secured on the top of your partner's butt so it doesn't slide down.

5. Pull the rope around to the front just under the hip, down between the legs, up over their butt, and meet that first rope with another Munter Hitch.

6. Take the free end and pull it up into the knot in the middle of the waist wrap, then cross over and up.

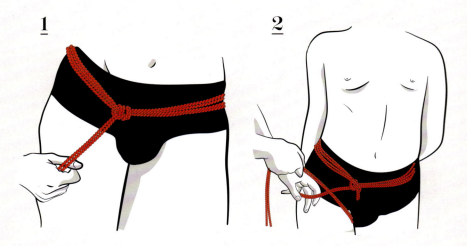

108   THE BONDAGE PLAYBOOK

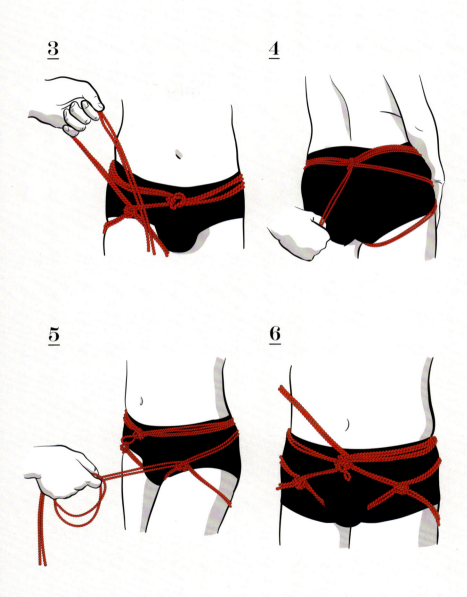

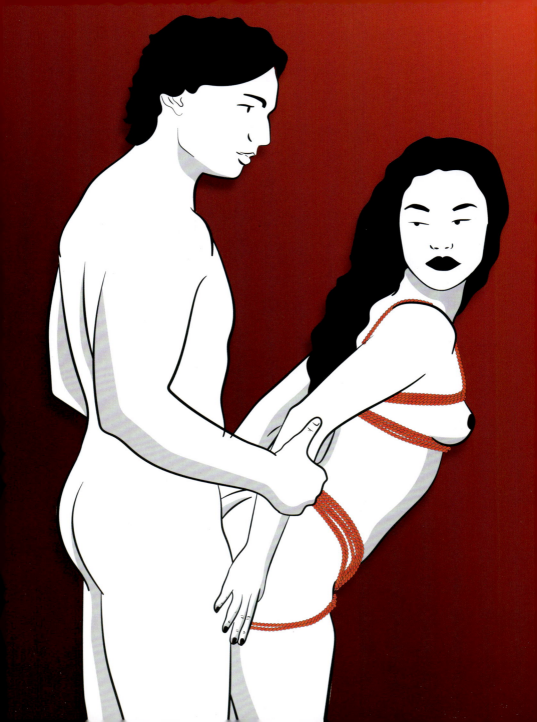

The Infinity

Build on the Beginner Sex Harness Hip Tie (page 106) with a harness to highlight your partner's breasts or chest muscles. This also involves a weaving technique.

HOW TO DO IT:

1. Make a wrap around the chest, bringing the rope up and over one breast or pectoral muscle.

2. Change direction, coming around the front to go up and over the other breast or muscle.

3. Repeat, building on your foundation by weaving in and out as you cross over each new wrap.

4. When you have about 3 feet (1 m) left of rope, split the pair in your hand and come up and over the shoulders to the front.

5. Weave it down into the top wraps and back up over the shoulder to keep the ropes from sliding off.

6. Return to the original knot in the back, taking care to keep it neat and tie it off. You can add a bow if you like!

1 **2**

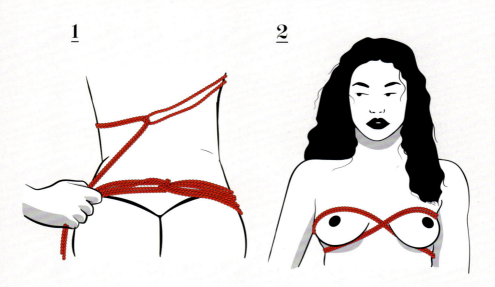

THE BONDAGE PLAYBOOK

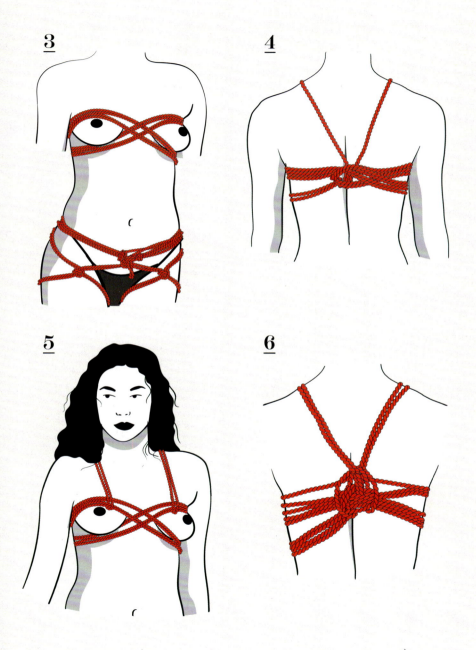

Karada

This tie uses a series of knots to form diamond patterns across the body, a technique typically known in the West as a Karada. It's a decorative tie used to highlight your partner's body.

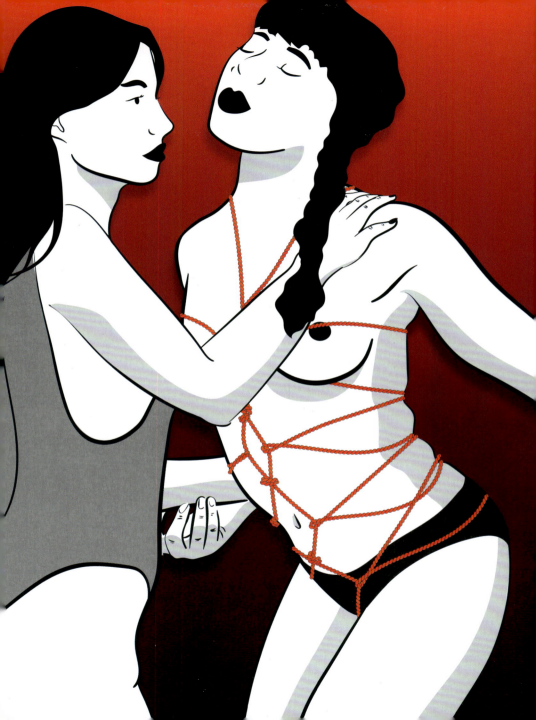

HOW TO DO IT:

1. Fold the rope in half and tie a simple Overhand Knot about a foot down at the bight end.

2. Slip the rope over your partner's head so the knot sits on the back of their neck. The loop will be hanging down their back and the two ends of the rope split over their shoulders. Make sure the rope lies extremely loosely around their neck. Bring the two ends of the rope back together in front of the body and create a new knot between the collarbone and nipples.

3. Make a series of knots about 6 inches (15 cm) apart all the way down the front of the body. Bring the rope between the legs and up the back, pulling the ends through the first loop that is hanging down your partner's back.

4. Split the ends of the doubled-over rope and take them under the arms, cross them over and then under the rope lying vertically between the top two knots. Pull on the two ends of the rope and the vertical rope should separate, creating the diamond shape.

5. Wrap around the back and come back to make another diamond between the next two knots.

6. Repeat the process, coming all the way down the body. Tie off and enjoy the visual feast you have created.

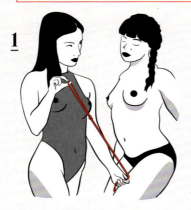

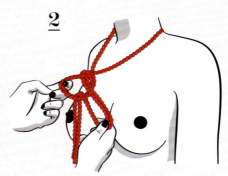

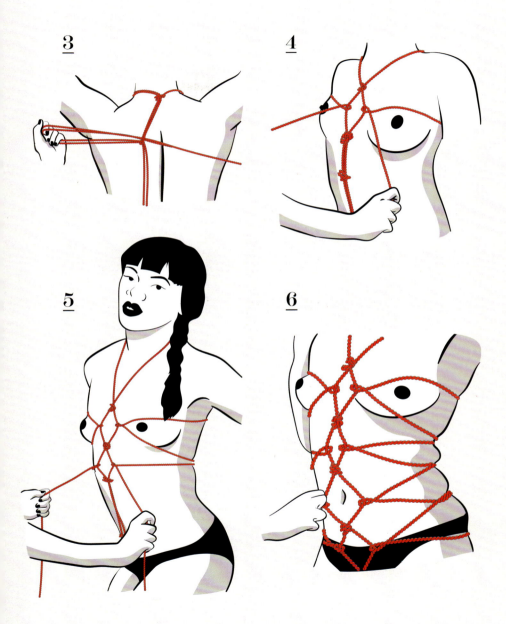

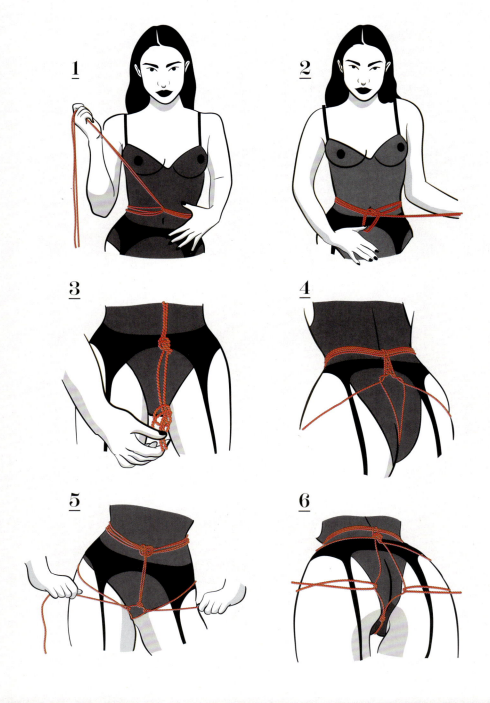

Ass Opener

Like the Self-Serve Chest Tie (page 77), this is a knot you tie yourself to adorn yourself for your partner. Again, never do any sort of bondage on your own—you'll need to have someone with you while you tie. Once tied, you can give your partner a little show by playing with yourself with your hands or a toy, or teasing your partner before letting them ravish you. This is generally a knot for people with vulvas (there's a knot right on the clit which can be a turn on for some), but if you have a penis, just shift it until it feels comfortable. Because the back is opened, it's great for anal sex.

HOW TO DO IT:

1. Make a few wraps around the body ending in the front.

2. Make a simple knot around the whole series of wraps and tighten it. The free end should be hanging down in front of your groin.

3. Make two knots in the length of the rope. The lower knot should hang either right in front of the clit or just below it if you have a vulva, or wherever feels comfortable if you have a penis.

4. Pull the rope up between the legs to the back, then through the waist wraps and make a knot. Pull the ends to open the back.

5. Take each end and bring it around the front, pulling through the doubled rope across your groin, tugging it to open a space.

6. Pass the ropes around your back and bring it over and under the back ropes so you're spreading them apart. Tie off in the front around your waist and enjoy!

TAKING IT FURTHER

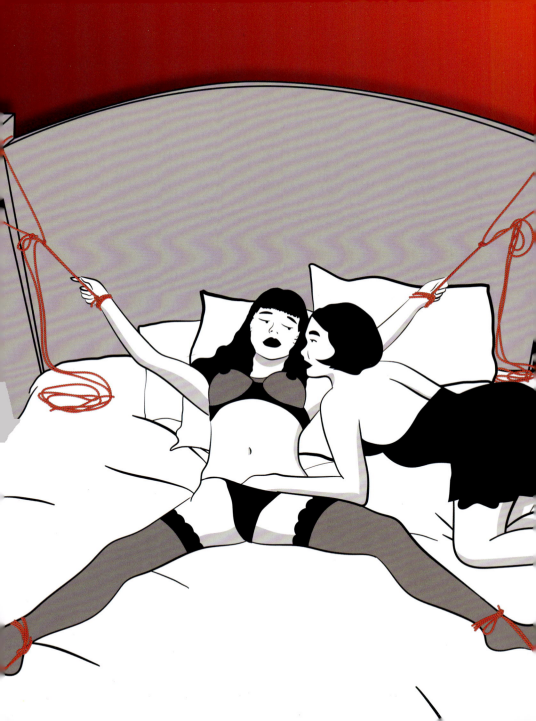

Trucker's Hitch

Use this for binding your partner so they're spread-eagled to the bed. The hitch allows you to retighten the knot anytime, if needed. It works well for Dom/sub scenarios. You can edge your partner, refusing to let them orgasm until you decide they can, or just have your way with them. For a variation you can use this same technique but have your partner face down or tie their legs up to the headboard post.

HOW TO DO IT:

1. Start with a Bula Bula (page 20) around the ankle.
2. Make a slipknot just below the toe of the foot.
3. Wrap the free end of the rope around a bedpost and come back up. Feed the loose end of the rope through the loop of the slipknot and pull the leg snug. The loop will act just like a pully. Pinch the first loop to hold it in place for the next step, making a loop just below it.
4. Pull a 12 inch (30.5 cm)-long loop through.
5. Tug the rope to make it as snug as you'd like.
6. The slipknot allows you to quickly pull the loose end if you need to free your partner, or retighten the rope as you go. Repeat the process on your partner's remaining leg and their two arms.

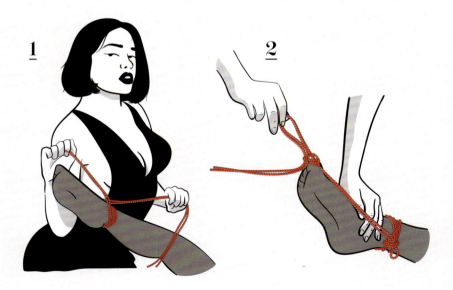

THE BONDAGE PLAYBOOK

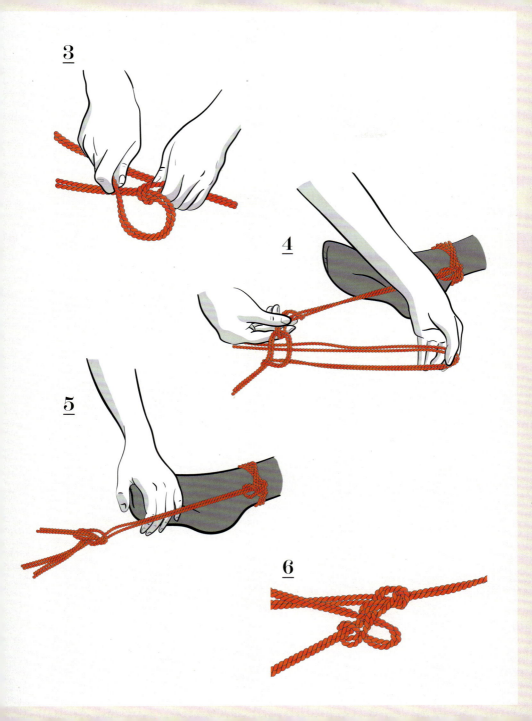

Rope Corset

Make a full-on corset using just rope. It looks elaborate but it's really an easy pattern that you repeat to create the look. Just make sure you start with enough rope to do the job.

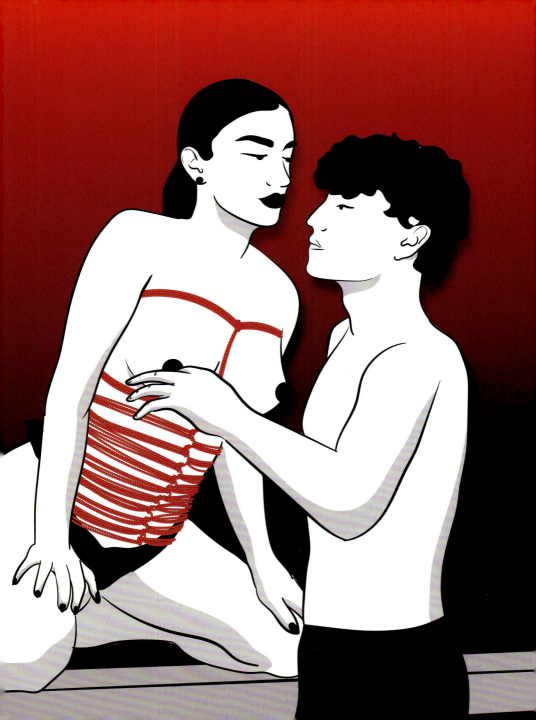

HOW TO DO IT:

1. Fold the rope in half to create a bight end. Wrap the rope once around the back to the front, keeping it above the breasts. Feed the loose end through the loop.

2. Bring the rope straight down between the breasts and hold it there while you come around the back to the front again.

3. Pass the loose end through the vertical rope and come around the back again, making a full wrap.

4. Now come through the loop in the front, reversing the way you came.

5. Pull the rope down and repeat steps 2 to 4.

6. Build the corset all the way down by repeating the same pattern. If you run out of rope, add more using the Joining Rope technique (page 28).

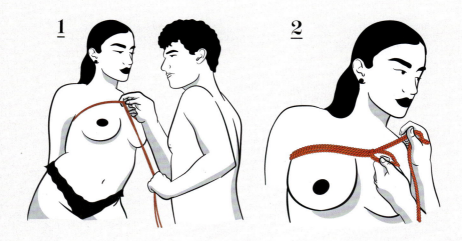

126   THE BONDAGE PLAYBOOK

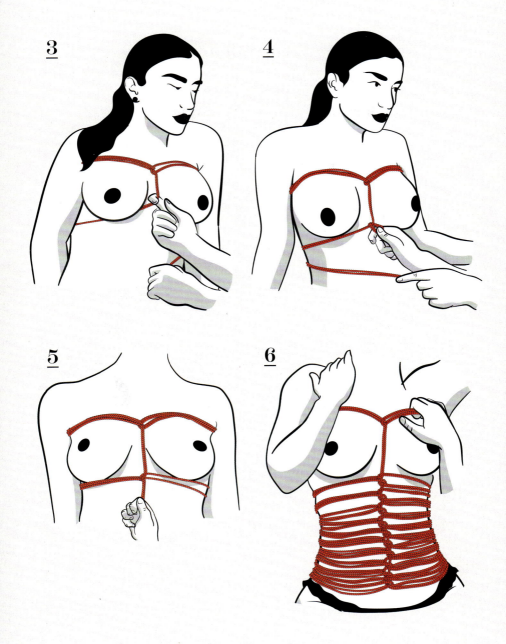